NEW WAYS TO CARE FOR OLDER PEOPLE

Evan Calkins, MD, is a graduate of Harvard Medical School, with house staff training at Johns Hopkins Hospital and the Massachusetts General Hospital and a fellowship in biochemistry at Harvard Medical School, Dr. Calkins became attracted, early in his career, to the need for applying the results of basic biomedical research in the care of patients with chronic illness. He accepted an appointment as a member and later director of the Arthritis Unit at the Massachusetts General Hospital. In 1961 he was appointed co-chairman and, later, chairman of the Department of Medicine at the State University of New York at Buffalo. In 1997 he resigned this position to become founding director of the Division of Geriatrics/ Gerontology at this University, the seventh such division in this country. Together with Harvard University, University of Michigan, and University of Southern California at Los Angeles, SUNY Buffalo was selected as the site for the development of one of four prototype geriatric education centers. During his 12-year leadership of the division, Dr. Calkins was responsible for recruiting and training what was, at that time, 10% of the fellowship-trained geriatricians in the country. In 1990, Dr. Calkins accepted appointment as Senior Physician and Coordinator, Geriatrics Programs, in HealthCarePlan, a not-for-profit HMO. A former member of the Advisory Council of the National Institute of Aging, Dr. Calkins is a Master of the American College of Physicians and the American College of Rheumatology, a Fellow and Past-Chair of the Clinical Medical section of the Gerontological Society of America, and a Fellow of the American Geriatric Society.

Chad Boult, MD, MPH, is an associate professor and the research director of the University of Minnesota Center on Aging. For the past decade, he has designed, implemented, studied and reported the effects of emerging systems of health care for older populations, including case management, rehabilitation, geriatric evaluation and management (GEM), and team care of nursing home residents. In 1993, he developed a widely used instrument for identifying older persons with a high probability of repeated hospital admissions (the P_{ra}). He teaches and practices geriatric medicine and frequently lectures and consults with health care organizations and academic institutions. With his wife (a geriatrician/historian) and three children, he lives in St. Paul.

Edward H. Wagner, MD, MPH, is a graduate of Princeton University and the School of Medicine, State University of New York at Buffalo, Dr. Wagner undertook his internship and residency in Internal Medicine at the affiliated hospitals, SUNY Buffalo. Between internship and residency years, he served in the Military Core of the Army of the United States, one year of which was spent in Vietnam. In 1983, he became Founding Director of the Center for Health Studies at Group Health Cooperative of Puget Sound, and Professor in the Department of Health Services in the University of Washington's School and Community Medicine. His research, focused on issues of preventive care, chronic disease management, and the design and evaluation of innovative patterns of health care delivery, is summarized in 177 publications in reviewed medical journals, and numerous invited lectureships, chapters, and books. He is currently Director at the MacColl Institute for Health Care Innovation, Group Health Cooperative, and Professor, University of Washington School of Public Health and Community Medicine.

James T. Pacala, MD, MS, is an associate professor in the Department of Family Practice and Community Health at the University of Minnesota Medical School. He received his undergraduate degree from Carleton College, an MD from the University of Rochester, and an MS in Chronic Disease Epidemiology from Brown University. He has served as the Medical Director for the University of Minnesota Senior Health Center for the past 3 years. Dr. Pacala has performed extensive research in the care of older adult populations, focusing on health risk screening, case management, and prevention. In addition to his research, Dr. Pacala teaches geriatric medicine to medical students, residents, and fellows.

NEW WAYS TO CARE FOR OLDER PEOPLE

Building Systems Based on Evidence

EVAN CALKINS, MD

CHAD BOULT, MD, MPH

EDWARD H. WAGNER, MD, MPH

JAMES T. PACALA, MD, MS

Editors

 Springer Publishing Company

The authors would like to thank Jennifer Weuve, BA, for her persistence, good humor, and fine literary skills in coordinating and copyediting the manuscript for this book.

Springer Publishing Company, Inc.
536 Broadway
New York, NY 10012-3955

Cover design by Margaret Dunin
Acquisitions Editor: Helvi Gold
Production Editor: Kathleen Kelly

99 00 01 02 03 / 6 5 4 3 2

Library of Congress Cataloging-in-Publication-Data

New ways to care for older people : building systems based on
   evidence in managed care / edited by Evan Calkins . . . [et al.].
      p.   cm.
   Includes bibliographical references and index.
   ISBN 0-8261-1220-X
   1. Aged—Medical care.   2. Aged—Medical care—United States.
I. Calkins, Evan.
RA564.8.N5   1998
362.1'9897—dc21   98-38606
                                                          CIP

Printed in the United States of America

Contents

Preface

It is indeed satisfying to see the development and publication of this book aimed at bringing the best of current knowledge to bear on the challenges in caring for older persons. The coeditors and the highly qualified authors of chapters recognize that our aging population presents us with the widest possible range of needs and opportunities, from maintenance of good health and independence to integrated continuing care and quality of life in the face of multiple coexistent health and social problems. They address this broad agenda responsibility through use of sound, evidence-based information. The sequence of chapters not only helps a reader find relevant information on his or her immediate question on care for a given patient but also brings attention to the range of possibilities for caring settings and approaches that might also be relevant.

T. FRANKLIN WILLIAMS

Foreword

The evolution of geriatric care is a story of cups. As one reads through the chapters in this book, it is hard not to recognize that a great deal of innovative ideas have been developed and a growing body of evidence has amassed about better systems of care. Seen in this light, the geriatric cup is more than half full. It seems evident, however, that even more can be done. The ultimate value of many of these innovations, especially when integrated into large systems, remains to be proven. The testing will be conducted in stages. The first question to be addressed is whether doing what is recommended will make a substantial difference to health. The next issue is whether the gains achieved will be worth their cost. Here the geriatric cup is emptier; the empirical basis to support many geriatric recommendations is still underdeveloped. Indeed, the slip between the cup of promise and the lip of practical implementation may be serious.

In a sense, the developments in the care of chronic disease come at a propitious time. The management of chronic disease (an infelicitous term that unfortunately implies managing disease instead of helping people with these afflictions) is central to health care efforts because chronic disease lies at the heart of contemporary health care. The vast majority of the effort and money devoted to medical care goes toward chronic disease in one manifestation or another (Hoffman, Rice, & Sung, 1996). Seen in this light, it is incredible that the health care industry is still acting as if it were in the acute care business. The present fragmented system (or nonsystem) of care is technologically sophisticated but organizationally inept. Huge efforts are expended on diagnosis and treatment without coordination, sometimes resulting in expensive duplication of efforts, and frequently losing efficiency because information is inadequately, incorrectly, or belatedly transferred among the many players involved. The emphasis on the management of disease must find room for equal attention to patient-centered care. The enthusiasm for establishing clinical protocols must acknowledge the difficulties of defining correct actions in a context of multiple interacting problems. New *modi operandi* are urgently needed. The systems discussed in this volume point the way to some of those sorely needed innovations.

Not only is the focus of medical care shifting—so too is its context. The escalating costs of care have been blamed on the aging of the population, but they are attributable mainly to the logarithmic growth in the use of medical technology (Advisory Council on Social Security, 1991). Whatever the cause, the demand for cost controls has led to new efforts to constrain the medical care system. The banner under which many of the efforts fly is managed care. The central element of modern managed care is often a deliberate effort to constrain expenditures. In the best case, careful deliberation is given to selecting the treatments or interventions that are likely to yield the best results at the lowest cost. Managed care could prove a boon for geriatrics and for the management of chronic disease because it has the potential to take the long view. The benefits need not be immediate; investments in more intensive management may be economically justified if they can be shown to yield subsequent benefits—expressed in terms of better health, as well as lower costs. So far, a few geriatric innovations have passed this test. Some forms of comprehensive geriatric assessment and home care have demonstrated reductions in the use of institutional care (Stuck, Siu, Wieland, & Rubenstein, 1993). Other innovations offer some indications that they too will be shown to be cost-effective, especially in a longitudinal context.

Managed care could provide an environment supportive of the integration of many of these innovations. Its structure could facilitate coordination and oversight to end the border disputes between professions and institutions about who has the rights to various domains of diagnosis and treatment. Coordinated interdisciplinary teams have the potential to reduce redundancy and to integrate the hitherto disparate components of health care.

One important adjunct in such a struggle is the constructive use of information systems. Information may prove to be one of the most potent technologies in the drive to improve the care of older people with chronic conditions. Information systems can impose structure on data collection and diagnostic efforts. They can assist clinicians to advance logically and comprehensively. They can monitor progress toward defined clinical goals and indicate when adequate progress is not being achieved. They can assure that all pertinent parties are kept abreast of developments and changes in patients' status. Investments in information infrastructures are more feasible in large organizations where the costs can be spread over thousands of encounters per day. Corporate enthusiasm for such investments in information technology would be intensified by evidence that improved monitoring and communication create dividends in better outcomes.

The picture with managed care is far from rosy, however. Most managed care is not geriatrically oriented. Business as usual is still the norm. In the short run, there are more short-term financial gains to be made by racheting down than by building up. As discussed in Chapter 20, the challenge for society will be to create incentives that will harness and direct the potential good that managed care can do. Before that scenario can exist, policy makers must see clearly what is possible. Some of the material in this volume offers a glimpse into that world of the possible, but it is a cautious glance. By emphasizing the importance of building systems based on evidence, the authors have focused on extant technologies, but much more innovation remains to be done.

Readers of these chapters may find their appetites more whetted than satisfied. So many possibilities loom. So much needs to be tested. The question is where to begin. There is no simple basis for making such a choice. It is more a question of personal preference. Some are drawn to prevention and health promotion, a strategy that addresses the largest numbers and promises the most positive long-term effects. While it would be almost sacrilegious to disparage efforts at health promotion, such a fixation can be dangerous, especially in the context of managed care. It is much too easy to distract both patients and overseers into concentrating their attention on such activities and thus to overlook the deficiencies in other areas. The ultimate test of managed care will not be how it handles healthy people. Indeed it has every incentive to actively recruit healthy customers. The real test of managed care will be how it handles the sick. Hence, the place to begin in establishing the efficacy of innovations is with those who are sick, especially those who have complex problems. Preventive efforts are best directed at avoiding iatrogenic problems and reducing the transition from disease to disability.

The programs described herein offer a menu of opportunities. Some observers might marvel at how far we have come. Others will be struck by how much remains to be accomplished. At the risk of equivocating, I would urge us move quickly but carefully. Speed is needed because medical care is riding the back of a galloping beast. Changes in the organization, financing, and delivery of health care are occurring so rapidly that some good ideas not tested quickly are abandoned in favor of the next fad. At the same time the consequences of excessive zeal for unproven ideas are enormous. Unfortunately we are living in a schizophrenic era. The current climate features simultaneously both a hunger for new ideas and a skepticism about them. We need prompt evaluations of the effectiveness of new systems of care, where the outcomes are expressed in terms that appeal to clinicians, administrators, and patients alike. This is a tall order.

ROBERT L. KANE

REFERENCES

Advisory Council on Social Security. (1991). *Critical issues in American health care delivery and financing policy* (pp. 303–313). Washington, D.C.: Author.

Hoffman, C., Rice, D., & Sung, H.-Y. (1996). Persons with chronic conditions: their prevalence and costs. *Journal of the American Medical Association, 276,* 1473–1479.
Stuck, A. E., Siu, A. L., Wieland, G. D., & Rubenstein, L. Z. (1993). Comprehensive geriatric assessment: a meta-analysis of controlled trials. *Lancet, 342,* 1032–1036.

Introduction

The rapid aging of the population and its impact on health care providers and systems are no longer the theoretical concerns of futurists and academicians. Most health systems and many clinicians are frantically searching for ways to respond to the greater clinical demands without going bankrupt. For those systems and providers that have taken action, the most common innovations are targeting, assessment, and case management. This catechism is now being played out in hundreds of health systems across the country. Will it succeed? Will it make care more relevant and effective for our growing population of older people?

The importance of targeting is self-evident given the heterogeneity of older people and their health care needs. But targeting should differentiate subgroups who will benefit from different arrays of clinical and supportive services, not simply divide the senior population into two groups—a small one that gets special attention and a larger one left to fend for itself.

Assessments that focus on past utilization and fail to evaluate quality of life, function, and physiologic reserve will limit a system's ability to prevent disability and maintain independence. Case management, whose primary goal is reducing utilization, may change the location of care, that is, from inpatient to outpatient, at the expense of its quality.

In this book, we focus on the evidence on interventions that improve outcomes and reduce costs in older adults. This evidence, largely derived from randomized, clinical trials, suggests that organizations seeking to improve the health of older populations should address

- the full gamut of health needs of older persons, from the prevention of illness to dignified dying
- the ability of today's providers to meet these needs
- all of the settings in which older persons receive their care
- the full array of successful innovations described in the following chapters

Scientifically based geriatric care will not just carve out a small group for special attention. It will understand and address the needs of the entire population of older people: the frequent transitions from one health state to another, the crucial role of self-management, the interactions between the physical and social influences on health, the devastating effects of deconditioning, and the ever-present threat of iatrogenesis. Promoting the creation of systems capable of addressing these various needs in a humane, scientifically sound, consistent, and integrated way is the goal of this book. It will take more than targeting, assessment, and case management.

We systematically examine the evidence of what works and what doesn't in improving health outcomes among the full range of older people from triathletes to those near the end of life. While evidence suggests that some interventions that improve health do, in fact, also reduce health care costs or are cost neutral, our focus remains firmly fixed on improving health outcomes, not on reducing cost at the possible expense of health. Our perspective throughout the book is on older people rather than on the facilities, institutions, or professionals from which they receive care. We attempt to describe optimal systems that care for older people as they progress from robust health, where prevention is the dominant concern, through chronic illness, increasing dependency, and death, where maintenance of personhood and control are central.

Each chapter describes and evaluates those interventions and practice innovations that, in well-designed evaluations, have improved outcomes. While improvements in the prevention and therapy of important geriatric conditions such as influenza, congestive heart failure, myocardial infarction, and systolic hypertension have made substantial contributions to the reduced morbidity and mortality of older Americans, specific clinical conditions are not the focus of the book. Rather, we focus on changes in the organization, delivery, evaluation, and financing of care that are most likely to allow greater proportions of older adults to receive the best available treatments and the support needed to help them sustain their health and independence.

Our perspective is population-based, a term that, to some, connotes impersonal, cookie-cutter care. In our view, however, the term reminds us that optimal patient care is proactive, reaching out to all those in a population who need services, not waiting to react only to those who appear in the waiting or emergency room. It is not adequate to immunize against influenza and pneumonia only those who happen to visit a clinic during autumn months, to assess the mental status only of those complaining of memory lapses, or to allow chronically ill patients to become lost to follow-up. Adequate patient care means initiating the action, reminding patients that immunizations or follow-up are needed, and assessing cognitive function and other critical conditions that are likely to be underreported. Initiating the action requires that a system have responsibility for a defined population, information about the population, and an array of effective, proactive interventions, some of which are as simple as postcard reminders or practice-initiated telephone calls. While capitation aids population-based care by defining an enrolled population, it is by no means essential; many fee-for-service practices have identified their senior populations and developed clinical databases to assist with their management. Is population-based care incompatible with high-quality personalized care? The evidence suggests the opposite.

Our perspective is also evidence-based, another term in wide currency. Although we include few formal meta-analyses, we give priority to innovations that have proven successful in randomized clinical trials. Fortunately, many important geriatric care innovations—interdisciplinary home care, geriatric evaluation and management units, and disability prevention programs—have been evaluated rigorously, and data about their outcomes provide the core of most chapters and the basis for our recommendations. In some instances, the data and the resulting recommendations disagree with geriatric orthodoxy.

Our perspective is also patient-centered—organizing health related services around the needs of patients, rather than around the needs of institutions or providers. How does patient-centeredness manifest? Some of the interventions described occur in settings that may initially appear more attractive to patients than to their providers—the home, the senior center, or in group meetings. Others involve professionals whose primary job is to organize and coordinate the complex regimens of health care. As discussed in several chapters, evidence supports involving patients at the center of therapeutic decisions, treatment planning, care management, and end-of-life planning. Many of the successful innovations include concerted efforts to involve patients and their caregivers as active participants in decision-making and to pay explicit attention to their roles as managers of their illnesses and social needs. Patient-centeredness is not just to philosophy or an approach marketing; it is fundamental to improving health outcomes. Achieving it will require resources and commitment to change.

Readers will notice that the successful innovations we describe have tended either to create new systems of care or alter significantly older ones. They involve improvements such as the use of computers and computer data to identify, monitor, and communicate with patients and other caregivers. The integration of care between facilities and between health and social services is not left to chance, or to the patient, but to designated staff and communication systems. The new systems rely heavily on targeting, assessment, and case management but only as parts of an integrated system, not as separate services for the select. The success of many of the interventions described, in our view, results less from the constellation of activities chosen than from the manner with which these activities are stitched together into a coherent whole. The stitching is often a care or case manager who understands the clinical, social, and self-management issues and who works closely with primary and specialty providers to ensure sound and tailored treatment plans.

The book conveys the good news that there is now considerable positive evidence upon which to build more effective systems of care for older people. To incorporate these ideas into busy medical practice will be no mean task given the acute care orientation of most present clinical cultures and practice systems and the antipathy to geriatric care among some nongeriatricians. While major unanswered questions remain, the construction of scientifically sound, integrated systems able to meet the full needs of older populations is within reach, but only to those organizations, managers, and policymakers willing and able to engage in the major work of system change.

Contributors

Chad Boult, MD, MPH
Associate Professor
Department of Family Practice and
  Community Health
University of Minnesota School
  of Medicine
Minneapolis, MN

David C. Buchner, MD, MPH
Professor, Department of Health
  Services
School of Public Health and
  Community Medicine
University of Washington
Co-Director, Northwest Prevention
  Effectiveness Center
Seattle, WA

John Burton, MD
Professor of Medicine
Division of Geriatric Medicine
Francis Scott Key Medical Center
Baltimore, MD

Evan Calkins, MD
Emeritus Professor of Medicine
  and Family Medicine
State University of New York
  at Buffalo
Consultant in Geriatrics
HealthCarePlan and Promedicus
  Health Group
Buffalo, NY

Eric A. Coleman, MD, MPH
Robert Wood Johnson Clinical
  Scholar
University of Washington
Division of Geriatric Medicine
Harborview Medical Center
Seattle, WA

Karen Connors, RN
Director of Case Management
Healthcare Associates
Buffalo, NY

Amasa B. Ford, MD
Professor Emeritus of Epidemiology
  and Biostatistics
Associate Dean Emeritus of
  Geriatric Medicine
Case Western Reserve University
  School of Medicine
Cleveland, OH

George C. Halvorson
President & CEO
Health Partners
Minneapolis, MN
Senior Fellow, University of
  Missouri School of Business

Susan C. Hedrick, PhD
Associate Director
Center for Outcomes Research
  in Older Adults
Health Sciences Research and
  Development Program
VA Puget Sound Health Care
  System
Professor, Department of Health
  Services
School of Public Health and
  Community Medicine
University of Washington
Seattle, WA

**Deirdre Johnson, MB, BCH,
  MRC Psych., FRCPC**
Clinical Assistant Professor
Department of Psychiatry and
  Behavioral Medicine
Wake Forest University
Baptist Medical Center
Winston-Salem, NC

Robert Kane, MD
Minnesota Chair in Long-Term
  Care in Aging
Professor, School of Public Health
University of Minnesota
Minneapolis, MN

Andrew M. Kramer, MD
Research Director, Center on Aging
Associate Professor
Division of Geriatric Medicine
University of Colorado Health
  Sciences Center
Denver, CO

Bruce Leff, MD
Assistant Professor of Medicine
Johns Hopkins University School
  of Medicine
Assistant Professor of Health
  Policy and Management
Johns Hopkins University School
  of Hygiene and Public Health
Johns Hopkins Bayview
  Medical Center
Baltimore, MD

Harold S. Luft, PhD
Caldwell B. Esselystyn Professor
  of Medicine
Director, Institute for Health
  Policy Studies
University of California
San Francisco, CA

Robert McCann, MD
Assistant Professor of Medicine
University of Rochester
Rochester General Hospital
Rochester, NY

Chris Michalakes, DO
Assistant Professor of Clinical
  Emergency Medicine
School of Medicine and
  Biomedical Sciences
State University of New York
  at Buffalo
Clinical Chief
Emergency Medicine
Buffalo General Hospital
Buffalo, NY

Bruce Naughton, MD
Associate Professor of Clinical
  Medicine
SUNY at Buffalo
Buffalo, NY

James T. Pacala, MD, MS
Associate Professor
University of Minnesota
  Department of Family Practice
  and Community Health
Minneapolis, MN

Burton V. Reifler, MD, MPH
Professor and Chairman
Department of Psychiatry and
  Behavioral Medicine
Wake Forest University School
  of Medicine
North Carolina Baptist Hospital
Winston-Salem, NC

David B. Reuben, MD
Chief, Division of Geriatrics
Director, Multicampus Program
  in Geriatric Medicine and
  Gerontology
Professor of Medicine
University of California at
  Los Angeles
Los Angeles, CA

John F. Schnelle, PhD
Professor of Medicine
Director of Borun Center for
  Gerontological Research
University of California at
  Los Angeles Jewish Home
  for the Aging
Reseda, CA

Thomas vonSternberg, MD
Associate Medical Director,
  Geriatrics
Health Partners
Associate Clinical Professor
Department of Family Practice and
  Community Health
University of Minnesota
Minneapolis, MN

Michael VonKorff, MD
Senior Investigator
Center for Health Studies
Group Health Cooperative
  of Puget Sound
Seattle, WA

Edward H. Wagner, MD, MPH
Director, MacColl Institute for
  Healthcare Innovation
Group Health Cooperative
  of Puget Sound,
Professor, School of Public Health
  and Community Medicine
University of Washington
Seattle, WA

William G. Weissert, PhD
Professor and Chair
Department of Health
  Management and Policy
School of Public Health
Senior Research Scientist
Institute of Gerontology
University of Michigan
Ann Arbor, MI

T. Franklin Williams, MD
Professor of Medicine, Emeritus
University of Rochester
VA Distinguished Physician
Monroe Community Hospital
Rochester, NY

I

When the Older Person Is Healthy and Independent

*I*t was not very long ago that scientists, clinicians, and the public believed that the decline in function associated with aging was inevitable. Researchers developed elaborate formulas for predicting future decrepitude, clinicians hung crepe, and well-meaning friends and family encouraged seniors to take it easy and enjoy life. Landmark gerontologic research showed that while the average physiologic capacity of a group of older people declined over time, many individuals within the group evidenced minimal or no decline. Further work suggested that these "successful" seniors had lived different lifestyles than those showing more typical decline.

Epidemiologists then began to look for other behavioral or medical characteristics that would predict which older adults would lose mobility and function and, ultimately, their independence. Studies of a variety of senior populations have demonstrated the predictive ability of a rather short list of characteristics led by inactivity and muscle weakness, followed by depression, overmedication, alcohol misuse, and, of course, the presence of chronic diseases. Even more recently, interventions directed at these predictors have been shown to reduce declines in function, losses of independence in activities of daily living (ADLs), and institutionalization, as well as prevention of falls. The core of these programs, as described in chapter 2, is physical activity.

Although the majority of seniors have one or more chronic conditions, there remain a host of opportunities to prevent disease or exacerbations of disease among older adults. Recent research has clarified the potential for disease prevention or early detection in older adults—the impact of risk factor reduction on coronary heart disease morbidity and mortality, the utility of smoking cessation, *the preventive roles of immunizations and aspirin or hormone replacement ther-apy, to name a few. These and other preventive opportunities for seniors are discussed in chapter 3.*

In most health systems, the vast majority of Medicare recipients will be highly functioning members of society. Keeping these people productive and indepen-dent will therefore remain a very high priority.

1

Prevention of Frailty

David M. Buchner

INTRODUCTION

The U.S. Preventive Services Task Force first published its *Guide to Clinical Preventive Services* in 1989 and followed with a second edition in 1996 (U.S. Preventive Services Task Force, 1996). This landmark effort rapidly became the premier reference source on the effectiveness of clinical preventive services, establishing evidence-based preventive care as the community standard.

The Task Force report shows how preventive care evolves throughout the life span. As we age, preventive care shifts emphasis from child safety and car seats, to bicycle helmets, to avoidance of drinking and driving, to cholesterol screening, and finally to flu shots (see chapter 2). Individual interventions have a different flavor depending on age. Smoking cessation programs for teenagers differ from programs for older adults (Kviz, Clark, Crittenden, Warnecke, & Freels, 1995). The recent Surgeon General's report on physical activity and health organizes its discussion of promoting physical activity according to age (U.S. Department of Health and Human Services, 1996).

One goal of preventive care is particularly important for older adults: the preservation of independence. This notion relates to the concept of compression of morbidity (Fries, 1980) and relates to public health objectives, as in *Healthy People 2000* (p. 447), to reduce the number of older adults who "have difficulty in performing two or more personal care activities" (U.S. Department of Health and Human Services, 1991). It relates to cultural values, such as that expressed in the adage that healthy aging involves "adding life to years, not adding years to life." It relates to the dread expressed by older adults at the possibility of leaving their homes to live in a nursing home. And it relates to the prevention of frailty.

One important cause of the loss of independence in older adults is an incompletely understood condition called "frailty." Limited scientific evidence suggests that integrating selected preventive care recommendations and medical treatment recommendations into an intervention package (a multiple risk factor intervention) can prevent or delay the onset of frailty. Although the evidence is incomplete and still accumulating, we can reasonably adopt an integrated approach to prevention of frailty now, because the main components of the package are each scientifically justifiable and because preventing loss of independence in older adults has enormous importance. The rationale for implementing these recommendations is enhanced by, but does not depend on, evidence of their efficacy in a frailty prevention program.

The first half of this chapter discusses the basic rationale and approach to frailty prevention, including a discussion of its definition and pathogenesis. Because a frailty prevention program is a new way to care for older adults, the second half of the chapter addresses possible concerns a provider or health care system might have upon considering whether to start such a program.

BUILDING A FRAILTY PREVENTION PROGRAM

What Is Frailty?

There is no scientific consensus on the definition and criteria for frailty. Consider the following two patients:

> *Patient 1, a 75-year-old man, was diagnosed with ischemic cardiomyopathy two years ago. He has stable congestive heart failure (CHF) treated with drugs. Still, he lifts weights and exercises regularly. He is hospitalized for surgery for benign prostatic hypertrophy (BPH). He walked safely around the hospital despite knee arthritis and needing to drag an IV pole with him. His surgeons prescribed a sedative drug to help him sleep in the hospital and discharged him after an uneventful hospital course.*

> *Patient 2 is similar to Patient 1 in some respects. He, too, is age 75 with congestive heart failure, knee arthritis, and BPH. But when hospitalized for surgery for BPH, he fell while walking to the bathroom with his IV pole. Pain medicines prescribed for injuries due to the fall caused him to become confused. After a few days of bed rest because of pain, he could barely get out of bed without assistance. He became incontinent. He left most of the food on his tray uneaten. After several days, the pain and confusion improved, but his gait was now unsteady and he was less mobile than before his hospital admission. His providers discharged him to a restorative care program in a nursing home, hopeful that he could return home after a few weeks of rehabilitation.*

Most would say that Patient 2 is frail and Patient 1 is not. Patient 2 appears vulnerable. He decompensates upon minor external stress—walking with an IV pole, taking a sedating drug, and remaining in bed a few days. He shows many signs and symptoms listed in textbook descriptions of frailty: weakness, fatigue, anorexia, decreased muscle mass, balance and gait abnormalities, marked deconditioning, and falls (Fried, 1994). In contrast, minor external stressors do not affect Patient 1.

A Framework for Understanding Frailty

A comparison of all the proposed definitions of frailty is beyond the scope of this chapter. Instead, we first provide a working definition. Then, after further describing frailty and its measurement, we present a framework for understanding disability.

In this chapter, frailty is

> best regarded as a condition or syndrome which results from a multi-system reduction in reserve capacity to the extent that a number of physiological systems are close to, or past, the threshold of symptomatic clinical failure. As a consequence, the frail person is at increased risk of disability and death from minor external stresses. (Campbell & Buchner, 1997)

The frameworks for understanding this and other definitions of frailty are the models used in the book *Disability in America* (Pope & Tarlov, 1991) and by the World Health Organization ICIDH (International Classification of Impairment, Disability, and Handicap) (Chamie, 1990). These models relate fundamental pathophysiologic changes in a person's ability to manage in various environments. The causes of disability (etiologic agents) operate on four levels:

- *Pathology* (disease) occurs at the cell and tissue level (e.g., the presence of lung cancer cells, atrophy of islet cells in the pancreas).
- *Impairment* (physiologic impairment) occurs at the organ and organ system level (e.g., reduced cardiac output, bone density, muscle strength, and creatinine clearance).
- *Functional limitations* occur at the level of the whole person (e.g., difficulty with simple movements and walking).
- *Disability* occurs at the level of the person-environment interaction. The environment encompasses both physical and social factors. A person in a wheel chair is not disabled if there is a ramp but is disabled if stairs provide the only entrance to the building.

Frailty, as a disabling process, has effects that are measurable at each level of this framework. Definitions can be understood in terms of which levels of the model are used to define and measure frailty.

Pathology.   The number and type of chronic diseases have been used to identify frail adults (MacAdam, Capitman, Yee, & Prottas, 1989; Pawlson, 1988), but this approach is least useful in defining and measuring frailty, because the pathophysiologic effects of common diseases like hypertension or diabetes vary so widely. In the example above, note that the two patients actually have the same chronic diseases, yet one is frail and the other is not.

Physiologic Impairment.   The working definition focuses on measuring frailty by assessing physiologic capacities.

Functional Limitations.   Geriatric medicine has long emphasized the importance of assessing functional limitations. Some authors regard tests of functional limitations as markers of frailty (Weiner, Duncan, Chandler, & Studenski, 1992), but tests of functional limitations are not specific to the cause of the limitation and so are not ideal for distinguishing frail from nonfrail adults. For example, a frail adult and a healthy adult with severe hip pain may walk at the same speed.

Disability.   Several definitions of frailty (including the one above) emphasize the person-environment interaction and the ability to perform the practical and social activities of daily living (Bortz, 1993; Brown, Renwick, & Raphael, 1995; Rockwood, Fox, Stolle, Robertson, & Beattie, 1994). This type of definition is broad and does not distinguish the concepts of frailty and disability.

Multilevel Definitions.   At least one study defined frailty as a combination of measures across all four levels (Speechley & Tinetti, 1991). Multilevel definitions of frailty will probably become more common.

Reducing the Rate of Loss of Physiologic Capacity

From the working definition, it follows that frailty is prevented by ensuring that key organ systems maintain adequate physiologic capacity. Since the relationship between physiologic capacity and functional limitations and disability is nonlinear (Buchner, Larson, Wagner, Koepsell, & de Lateur, 1996; Schwartz & Buchner, 1994), preventive interventions should attempt to preserve physiologic capacity in the range above the capacity required for usual daily activities. A working hypothesis posits that frailty results from failures in one or more of four types of physiologic capacities:

1. Endurance capacity is the capacity to sustain work. It depends upon maximum cardiac output, lung capacity, and the capacity of muscle to metabolize oxygen during contraction.

2. Musculoskeletal capacities involve joints (e.g., range of motion), muscles (e.g., strength), and bone (e.g., density).
3. Neurological capacities include the ability to assess the environment, make responsible judgments, and integrate visual, vestibular, and peripheral sensory clues.
4. Nutritional capacities include the ability to ingest and digest food and the capacity of the liver to synthesize albumin.

Ensuring adequate capacity during old age means reducing the rate of age-related loss of physiologic capacity by intervening on modifiable risk factors causing the loss. Evidence from epidemiologic studies has identified a number of potentially reversible risk factors for loss of mobility and function (Kaplan, 1997). At present, few interventions effectively restore capacity once it is lost. For example, smoking induces a loss in lung capacity. Stopping smoking will slow the rate of future loss, but lung tissue does not regenerate and restore capacity. A well-documented exception is physical activity, which increases physiologic capacities, such as endurance capacity and muscle strength, in older adults (Schwartz & Buchner, 1994). Table 1.1 depicts the relation between preventive interventions and physiologic capacities.

INTEGRATING PREVENTIVE INTERVENTIONS

Prevention programs often integrate the recommendations of the U.S. Preventive Services Task Force. Heart disease prevention programs focus on risk factors like high blood pressure, dietary fat, and smoking. Injury prevention programs focus on seat belts, bike helmets, and alcohol use while driving. Interventions designed to prevent frailty could also be combined into a single comprehensive program. What is the rationale and evidence for either separating or integrating these recommendations? We discuss the evidence from randomized trials first and then explain the rationale, using the trials as illustrations.

Limited scientific evidence supports the notion that a multiple risk factor approach can prevent disability and falls in older adults. Admittedly, these studies do not focus solely on preventing the clinical syndrome of frailty, but their essence is closely related to this goal. In particular, because the problems of frailty and falls are inter-related, studies of fall prevention provide information about prevention of frailty. The studies demonstrate the potential for preventing frailty, even though we do not know the optimal components of such a program.

In one population-based randomized trial, researchers reported that a multiple risk factor intervention in older adults reduced the 1-year incidence

TABLE 1.1 Examples of Effects of Prevention Care Intervention on Physiologic Capacities

Physiologic Capacities

Intervention	Endurance	Musculoskeletal	Neurological	Nutritional
Smoking cessation	Preserves lung and cardiac capacities by reducing lung damage and decreasing risk of heart disease		Preserves mental capacities by reducing risk of high blood pressure and stroke	May preserve lean body mass by improving caloric balance
Physical activity	Preserves/increases cardiac and muscle oxidative capacities	Preserves/increases muscle strength, joint range of motion, soft tissue flexibility, bone strength	Preserves mental capacities by reducing risk of high blood pressure and stroke, possible effect on neurophysiology	Preserves/increases lean body mass and decreases fat mass
Proper diet	Preserves cardiac capacities by reducing heart disease risk	Dietary calcium preserves bone strength	Preserves mental capacities by reducing obesity and decreasing risk of high blood pressure and stroke	Proper caloric balance preserves lean body mass and reduces fat mass

TABLE 1.1 Continued

Alcohol in moderation	Excessive alcohol can cause myopathy and cardiomyopathy	Excessive alcohol reduces bone strength, can cause myopathy, and increases injury risk	Excessive alcohol impairs mental capacities and can cause neuropathies	Excessive alcohol affects body composition and caloric intake
Treatment of depression	Preserves endurance by reducing psychomotor retardation	Preserves muscle strength by reducing psychomotor retardation		Preserves nutritional reserve by reducing anorexia
Reduce psychotropic drugs	Psychotropic drug use associated with reduction in endurance capacities		Psychotropic drugs can impair mental capacities	Psychotropic drugs can affect caloric intake
Treat undiagnosed disease	Many possible beneficial effects	Many possible beneficial effects	Many possible beneficial effects	Many possible beneficial effects

of decline in functional limitations from 13% to 7%; it also reduced fall rates from 37% to 27% (Wagner et al., 1994). The intervention addressed physical activity, hearing, vision, alcohol, psychotropic drug use, and home safety. The beneficial effects found at 1-year follow-up had dissipated by the 2-year follow-up evaluation, possibly because interventions occurred only in the first year.

Other researchers reported that a multiple risk factor intervention reduced the incidence of falls in a community population with fall risk factors (Tinetti et al., 1994). The interventions addressed the risk factors of psychotropic drug use, polypharmacy, muscle weakness, poor balance, poor gait, poor transfers, and postural hypotension. The intervention group had a 35% incidence of falls, compared with a 47% incidence in the social visit control group. A study involving environmental modification, recommendations about physical activity, and counseling about appropriate behavior also reported a reduction in falls (Hornbrook et al., 1994).

Another study examined annual in-home comprehensive geriatric assessment of community adults age 75 or older (Stuck et al., 1995). After 3 years, 12% of the intervention group, as opposed to 22% of the control group, had a functional impairment; 4% of the intervention group, as opposed to 10% of the intervention group, lived in nursing homes. We can characterize the interventions in this study as both preventive care (promotion of physical activity, proper nutrition, home safety; screening of body weight, vision, hearing, affect, and cognition) and medical care (use of over-the-counter medications, use of aids and devices, compliance with medication regimens, management of incontinence).

Since our approach to frailty prevention involves scientifically justified individual interventions, the scientific rationale for a multiple risk factor reduction program relates to (1) the evidence of the effectiveness of multiple risk factor intervention approach, (2) whether risk factors cluster and interact, and (3) whether interventions interact.

The multiple risk factor approach recognizes that modest changes in several risk factors can substantially affect outcomes. The study by Tinetti illustrates the power of the approach. The average number of risk factors declined by 1.1 in the experimental group, but careful analysis suggested that this relatively modest reduction was sufficient to account for the group's observed 35% reduction in falls (Tinetti, McAvay, & Claus, 1996).

If risk factors cluster and interact, a multiple risk factor approach is more efficient and possibly more effective in practice. Risk factors apparently do cluster to an extent (Hulshof et al., 1992; Puccio, McPhillips, Barrett-Connor, & Ganiats, 1990; Schroll et al., 1996), though not in all settings (Chao & Zyzanski, 1990). The detection of interaction among risk factors requires large samples, so adequately powered studies are expensive and difficult to conduct (Nguyen et al., 1994).

The extent to which interventions to prevent frailty are synergistic is unclear. Depression causes inactivity by producing psychomotor retardation, and inactivity is a risk factor for depressive illness (North, McCullagh, & Tran, 1990). It seems logical to intervene simultaneously on both physical activity and depression. Interventions addressing poor gait, balance, strength, and transfers are also potentially synergistic (Tinetti et al., 1994). An intervention to improve gait is presumably enhanced by strength training, as strength is a determinant of gait. Even if interventions do not interact, we clinically infer that certain interventions complement each other, such as physical activity and nutrition interventions. A preventive program that combines related interventions may be more coherent to participants and hence more effective.

IMPLEMENTING POPULATION-BASED PREVENTION

Implementing population-based prevention involves synthesizing clinical medicine and public health approaches. A case study at an HMO identified several factors related to success (Thompson, Taplin, McAfee, Mandelson, & Smith, 1995):

- a population-based assessment of health problems using epidemiologic methods
- involvement of practitioners, including training practitioners to help patients change behavior
- a system-based approach to implementation, taking into account the strengths and weaknesses of practitioners, the health care system, and the community
- use of automated clinical information systems to routinely capture risk information
- evaluation by evidence-based criteria
- feedback to the practitioners and health care system of program outcomes

One example of a successful prevention program at the HMO was influenza immunization. By 1991, the HMO was immunizing 75% of its healthy older members and 85% of older members with chronic illnesses (Pearson & Thompson, 1994).

QUESTIONS AND ISSUES INVOLVING
FRAILTY PREVENTION

This discussion closely links frailty prevention to a model of frailty that emphasizes preserving physiologic reserve. What if a provider disagrees with the model?

This model is useful for understanding how prevention programs may prevent disability and frailty and for deciding which interventions to include in a program. Other models may also be useful. In any event, programs must adapt to their local setting, and several different approaches may be fairly consistent with a model. Of course, it is more important to ensure that a program is consistent with available scientific evidence than with a specific model.

Frailty prevention programs strongly resemble health promotion programs for older adults. Why is frailty prevention different?

One of the benefits of understanding the scientific basis for frailty is the recognition that a health promotion approach may be as or more important in preventing frailty than a medical disease management approach. But frailty prevention differs from general wellness programs in two important respects. A wellness program might follow the broad recommendation that adults obtain 30 minutes of moderate-intensity activity most days of the week (Pate et al., 1995) without specifying a type of activity. A frailty prevention program would focus on preserving physiologic capacities and necessarily include activities that promote endurance, strength, balance, and flexibility. Frailty prevention programs may also include the management of certain symptomatic diseases (e.g., depression).

What is the major limitation of existing research in frailty prevention?

Perhaps the major limitation with existing studies is their focus on relatively brief interventions. In attempting to slow the rate of loss of physiologic capacity, interventions operating over a period of years should have greater effects than relatively short-term interventions.

Which interventions should be considered?

Table 1.2 provides one possible list of interventions based on the recommendations of the U.S. Preventive Services Task Force (U.S. Preventive Services Task Force, 1996).

Is there a key intervention?

Physical activity is a promising intervention, as activity not only reduces the rate of physiologic loss but also increases several physiologic capacities (see Table 1.1). One review article cited positive effects of activity on lean body mass, fat mass, total body water, endurance capacity, maximal cardiac output, resting heart rate, blood pressure, baroreceptor function, muscle strength, bone strength, reaction time, depression, insomnia, appetite, fatigue, basal metabolic rate, glucose intolerance and diabetes, red

TABLE 1.2 Possible Interventions to Include in a Frailty Prevention Program

U.S. Preventive Services Task Force Recommendations for Adults Age 65+	Other Justifiable Interventions
Screening body weight	Evaluating adults with depressive symptoms
Screening vision	Evaluating adults with symptoms of dementia
Screening hearing	Screening to identify treatable, symptomatic, but undiagnosed illness
Screening for problem drinking	
Counseling to avoid alcohol use while driving, swimming, boating, etc.	
Counseling regarding caloric intake, fat, fruits and vegetables, calcium	
Counseling regarding physical activity	
Counseling to reduce risk of falls including home hazard assessment, medication adjustment, reducing polypharmacy, reducing sedative drug and psychotropic drug use	
Counseling for tobacco use	

blood cell mass, joint flexibility, fat metabolism, some aspects of the immune system, and probably also some aspects of cognition (Fiatarone & Evans, 1990). Physical activity is also important, because inactivity is so prevalent in older adults—only 20% of older adults attain recommended levels of activity (U.S. Department of Health and Human Services, 1996). Evidence is rapidly accumulating that regular physical activity prevents falls (e.g., Buchner et al., 1997; Province et al., 1995) and reduces functional limitations (e.g., Ettinger et al., 1997; Judge, Underwood, & Gennosa, 1993; Wallace et al., 1998).

What is known about the cost-effectiveness of prevention as it relates to frailty?

Of course, the criterion for implementing preventive care is not that it reduces costs. We purchase large amounts of expensive medical care, some of it of dubious value. We should be willing to pay for preventive care of proven value. Limited information on cost-effectiveness is available. In the Stuck study, the cost-effectiveness of the intervention was estimated at $46,000 for each year of disability-free life gained (Stuck et al.,

1995). In the Tinetti study, the intervention reduced hospital costs, with intervention subjects averaging $2,000 less in hospital costs (Rizzo, Baker, McAvay, & Tinetti, 1996). A study of a health promotion program in older adults involving self-care reported lower health care costs in the intervention group (Fries, Bloch, Harrington, Richardson, & Beck, 1993). And a study of an exercise program reported fewer outpatient visits and hospital days in adults who exercised (Buchner et al., 1997). There is epidemiologic evidence that older adults who experience functional decline have increased hospital use (Mor, Wilcox, Rakowski, & Hiris, 1994) and that seniors with risk factors for frailty (smoking, drinking, obesity, inactivity) have higher health care costs (Leigh & Fries, 1992).

Are there other reasons for implementing frailty prevention programs?

Some studies suggest that preventive care increases satisfaction with care (Schauffler & Rodriguez, 1994). Measures of the quality of preventive care are relatively easy to apply, as compared to measures of the quality of chronic disease care (Kerr, Mittman, Hays, Leake, & Brook, 1996). As the results of such quality measurements are made public (see chapter 15), health care plans with good preventive care may gain marketing advantages.

What is the role of the primary care provider?

The primary care provider probably should be involved in frailty prevention (Durham et al., 1991), but the role of provider counseling is still evolving. One study of provider counseling was disappointing (Burton, Paglia, German, Shapiro, & Damiano, 1995), whereas others that did not rely much on primary care providers (Stuck et al., 1995; Tinetti et al., 1994; Wagner et al., 1994) or that promoted self-care (Fries et al., 1993) were more successful. The U.S. Preventive Services Task Force finds insufficient evidence to recommend for or against the effectiveness of provider counseling in the areas of physical activity and fall prevention (U.S. Preventive Services Task Force, 1996), but it does recommend counseling in other areas.

Won't a frailty prevention program just attract adults who need prevention the least?

Health status is an inconsistent predictor of participation in research studies of prevention; participation may relate more to social habits and demands on people's time (Schweitzer et al., 1994; Wagner, Grothaus, Hecht, & LaCroix, 1991; Watkins & Kligman, 1993). One community wellness program (as opposed to a research study) for older adults in an HMO reported that the program attracted adults with lower mental and social health status (but similar physical health status) than the average HMO enrollee (Buchner & Pearson, 1989). On the other hand, participants in a major falls intervention trial tended to be in better health than nonparticipants (Pacala, Judge, & Boult, 1996). Participation also depends on the benefit structure as provided by a health plan (Jensen, Counte, & Glandon, 1992). If one believes that prevention programs attract healthier adults, then offering preventive care may be viewed as a marketing strategy.

What if no benefits can be found 1 year after implementing a prevention program?

One advantage of a frailty prevention program is that it focuses attention on the outcomes of greatest interest to older adults—functional ability and general health. While it may not be reasonable to expect a prevention program to produce measurable effects immediately, the successful efforts described above demonstrated beneficial effects in 1 to 3 years. Successful preventive care programs at HMOs (Thompson et al., 1995; Lawrence, 1991) result from a long-term commitment to prevention.

CONCLUSION

Frailty, or the reduction of important physiologic capacities, is a critical determinant of disability and loss of independence in older adults. Several randomized trials have demonstrated that multicomponent interventions are effective in reducing declines in function and falls without increasing health care costs, in fact reducing costs in some studies. The interventions all involve the detection of risk factors such as inactivity or polypharmacy and interventions directed at these factors. Exercise may be a critical element in programs designed to prevent frailty. Given their safety and low cost, the implementation of such programs should be strongly considered in most systems of geriatric care.

REFERENCES

Bortz, W. M. (1993). The physics of frailty. *Journal of the American Geriatrics Society, 41*, 1004–1008.

Brown, I., Renwick, R., & Raphael, D. (1995). Frailty: Constructing a common meaning, definition, and conceptual framework. *International Journal of Rehabilitation Research, 18*, 93–102.

Buchner, D. M., & Pearson, D. C. (1989). Factors associated with participation in a community senior health promotion program: A pilot study. *American Journal of Public Health, 79*, 775–777.

Buchner, D. M, Cress, M. E., de Lateur B. J., Esselman, P. C., Margherita, A. J., Price, R., & Wagner, E. H. (1997). The effect of strength and endurance training on gait, balance, fall risk, and health services use in community-living older adults. *Journal of Gerontology, 52A,* M209–M217.

Buchner, D. M., Larson, E. B., Wagner, E. H., Koepsell, T. D., & de Lateur, B. J. (1996). Evidence for a non-linear relationship between leg strength and gait speed. *Age and Ageing, 25,* 386–391.

Burton, L. C., Paglia, M. J., German, P. S., Shapiro, S., & Damiano, A. M. (1995). The effect among older persons of a general preventive visit on three health behaviors: Smoking, excessive alcohol drinking, and sedentary lifestyle: the Medicare Preventive Services Research Team. *Preventive Medicine, 24,* 492–497.

Campbell, A. J., & Buchner, D. M. (1997). Unstable disability and the fluctuations of frailty. *Age and Ageing, 2b,* 315–318.

Chamie, M. (1990). The status and use of the International Classification of Impairments, Disabilities and Handicaps (ICIDH). *World Health Statistics Quarterly, 43,* 273–280.

Chao, J., & Zyzanski, S. J. (1990). Prevalence of lifestyle risk factors in a family practice. *Preventive Medicine, 19,* 533–540.

Durham, M. L., Beresford, S., Diehr, P., Grembowski, D., Hecht, J. A., & Patrick, D. L. (1991). Participation of higher users in a randomized trial of Medicare reimbursement for preventive services. *Gerontologist, 31,* 603–606.

Ettinger, W. H., Jr., Burns, R., Messier, S. P., Applegate, W., Rejeski, W. J., Morgan, T., Shumaker, S., Berry, M. J., O'Toole, M., Monu, J., & Craven, T. (1997). A randomized trial comparing aerobic exercise and resistance exercise with a health education program in older adults with knee osteoarthritis: The Fitness Arthritis and Seniors Trial (FAST). *Journal of the American Medical Association, 277,* 25–31.

Fiatarone, M. A, & Evans, W. J. (1990). Exercise in the oldest old. *Topics in Geriatric Rehabilitation, 5,* 63–77.

Fried, L. P. (1994). Frailty. In W. R. Hazzard, E. L. Bierman, J. P. Blass, W. H. Ettinger, & J. B. Halter (Eds.), *Principles of geriatric medicine and gerontology* (3rd ed., pp. 1149–1156). New York: McGraw-Hill.

Fries, J. F. (1980). Aging, natural death, and the compression of morbidity. *New England Journal of Medicine, 303,* 130–135.

Fries, J. F., Bloch, D. A., Harrington, H., Richardson, N., & Beck, R. (1993). Two-year results of a randomized controlled trial of a health promotion program in a retiree population: The Bank of America Study. *American Journal of Medicine, 94,* 455–462.

Hornbrook, M. C., Stevens, V. J., Wingfield, D. J., Hollis, J. F., Greenlick, M. R., & Ory, M. G. (1994). Preventing falls among community-dwelling older persons: Results from a randomized trial. *Gerontologist, 34,* 16–23.

Hulshof, K. F., Wedel, M., Lowik, M. R., Kok, F. J., Kistemaker, C., Hermus, R. J., ten Hoor, F., & Ockhuizen, T. (1992). Clustering of dietary variables and other lifestyle factors. *Journal of Epidemiology and Community Health, 46,* 417–424.

Jensen, J., Counte, M. A., & Glandon, G. L. (1992). Elderly health beliefs, attitudes, and maintenance. *Preventive Medicine, 21,* 483–497.

Judge, J. O., Underwood, M., & Gennosa, T. (1993). Exercise to improve gait velocity in older persons. *Archives of Physical Medicine and Rehabilitation, 74,* 400–406.

Kaplan, G. A. (1997). Behavioral, social and socioenvironmental factors adding years to life and life to years. In T. Hickey, M. A. Speers, & T. R. Prohaska (Eds.), *Public health and aging* (pp. 37–52). Baltimore: Johns Hopkins University Press.

Kerr, E. A., Mittman, B. S., Hays, R. D., Leake, B., & Brook, R. H. (1996). Quality assurance in capitated physician groups: Where is the emphasis? *Journal of the American Medical Association, 276,* 1236–1239.

Kviz, F. J., Clark, M. A., Crittenden, K. S., Warnecke, R. B., & Freels, S. (1995). Age and smoking cessation behaviors. *Preventive Medicine, 24,* 297–307.

Lawrence, D. M. (1991). A provider's view of prevention approaches in a prepaid group practice. *Cancer, 67,* 1767–1771.

Leigh, J. P., & Fries, J. F. (1992). Health habits, health care use and costs in a sample of retirees. *Inquiry, 29,* 44–54.

MacAdam, M., Capitman, J., Yee, D., & Prottas, J. (1989). Case management for frail elders: The Robert Wood Johnson Foundations Program for Hospital Initiatives in Long-Term Care. *Gerontologist, 29,* 737–744.

Mor, V., Wilcox, V., Rakowski, W., & Hiris, J. (1994). Functional transitions among the elderly: Patterns, predictors, and related hospital use. *American Journal of Public Health, 84,* 1274–1280.

Nguyen, T. V., Kelly, P. J., Sambrook, P. N., Gilbert, C., Pocock, N. A., & Eisman, J. A. (1994). Lifestyle factors and bone density in the elderly: Implications for osteoporosis prevention. *Journal of Bone and Mineral Research, 9,* 1339–1346.

North, T. C., McCullagh, P., & Tran, Z. V. (1990). Effect of exercise on depression. *Exercise and Sport Science Reviews, 18,* 379–415.

Pacala, J. T., Judge, J. O., & Boult, C. (1996). Factors affecting sample selection in a randomized trial of balance enhancement: The FICSIT Study. *Journal of the American Geriatrics Society, 44,* 377–382.

Pate, R. R., Pratt, M., Blair, S. N., Haskell, W. L., Macera, C. A., Bouchard, C. Buchner, D., Ettinger, W., Heath, G. W., King, A. C., Kriska, A., Leon, A. S., Marcus, B. H., Morris, J., Paffenbarger, R. S., Patrick, K., Pollock, M. L., Rippe, J. M., Sallis, J., & Wilmore, J. H. (1995). Physical activity and public health: A recommendation from the Centers of Disease Control and Prevention and the American College of Sports Medicine. *Journal of the American Medical Association, 273,* 402–407.

Pawlson, L. G. (1988). Hospital length of stay of frail elderly patients. *Journal of the American Geriatrics Society, 36,* 202–208.

Pearson, D. C., & Thompson, R. S. (1994). Evaluation of Group Health Cooperative of Puget Sound's Senior Influenza Immunization Program. *Public Health Reports, 109,* 571–578.

Pope, A. M., & Tarlov, A. R. (1991). *Disability in America.* Washington, DC: National Academy Press.

Province, M. A., Hadley, E. C., Hornbrook, M. C., Lipsitz, L. A., Miller, J. P., Mulroco, C. D., Ory, M. G., Sattin, R. W., Tinetti, M. E., & Wolf, S. L. (1995). The effects of exercise on falls in elderly patients: A preplanned meta-analysis of the FICSIT trials. *Journal of the American Medical Association, 273,* 1341–1347.

Puccio, E. M., McPhillips, J. B., Barrett-Connor, E., & Ganiats, T. G. (1990). Clustering of atherogenic behaviors in coffee drinkers. *American Journal of Public Health, 80,* 1310–1313.

Rizzo, J. A., Baker, D. I., McAvay, G., & Tinetti, M. E. (1996).The cost-effectiveness of a multifactorial targeted prevention program for falls among community elderly persons. *Medical Care, 34,* 954–969.

Rockwood, K., Fox, R. A., Stolle, P., Robertson, D., & Beattie, B. L. (1994). Frailty in elderly people: An evolving concept. *Canadian Medical Association Journal, 150,* 489–493.

Schauffler, H. H., & Rodriguez, T. (1994). Availability and utilization of health promotion programs and satisfaction with health plan. *Medical Care, 32,* 1182–1196.

Schroll, K., Carbajal, A., Decarli, B., Martins, I., Grunenberger, F., Blauw, Y. H., de Groot, C. P. (1996). Food patterns of elderly Europeans: SENECA investigators. *European Journal of Clinical Nutrition, 50* (Supp. 2), S86–S100.

Schwartz, R. S., & Buchner, D. M. (1993). Exercise in the elderly: physiologic and functional effects. In W. R. Hazzard, E. L. Bierman, J. P. Blass, W. H. Ettinger, & J. B. Halter (Eds.), *Principles of geriatric medicine and gerontology* (3rd ed., pp. 91–105). New York: McGraw Hill.

Schweitzer, S. O., Atchison, K. A., Lubben, J. E., Mayer-Oakes, S. A., De Jong, F. J., & Matthias R. E. (1994). Health promotion and disease prevention for older adults: Opportunity for change or preaching to the converted? *American Journal of Preventive Medicine, 10,* 223–229.

Speechley, M., & Tinetti, M. (1991). Falls and injuries in frail and vigorous community elderly persons. *Journal of the American Geriatrics Society, 39,* 46–52.

Stuck, A. E., Aronow, H. U., Steiner, A., Alessi, C. A., Bula, C. J., Gold, M. N., Yuhas, K. E., Nisenbaum, R., Rubenstein, L. Z., & Beck, J. C. (1995). A trial of annual in-home comprehensive geriatric assessments for elderly people living in the community. *New England Journal of Medicine, 333,* 1184–1189.

Thompson, R. S., Taplin, S. H., McAfee, T. A., Mandelson, M. T., & Smith, A. E. (1995). Primary and secondary prevention services in clinical practice: Twenty years' experience in development, implementation, and evaluation. *Journal of the American Medical Association, 273,* 1130–1135.

Tinetti, M. E., Baker, D. I., McAvay, G., Claus, E. B., Garrett, P. Gottschalk, M., Koch, M. L., Trainor, K., & Horwitz, R. I. (1994). A multifactorial intervention to reduce the risk of falling among elderly people living in the community. *New England Journal of Medicine, 331,* 821–827.

Tinetti, M. E., McAvay, G., & Claus, E. (1996). Does multiple risk factor reduction explain the reduction in fall rate in the Yale FICSIT Trial? *American Journal of Epidemiology, 144,* 389–399.

U.S. Department of Health and Human Services. (1991). *Healthy People 2000: National health promotion and disease prevention objectives.* (DHHS Publication No. PHS 91-50212). Washington, DC: U.S. Government Printing Office.

U.S. Department of Health and Human Services. (1996). *Physical activity and health: A report of the surgeon general.* Atlanta: U.S. Department of Health and Human Services, Center for Disease Control and Prevention, National Center for Chronic Disease Prevention and Health Promotion.

U.S. Preventive Services Task Force. (1996). *Guide to clinical preventive services,* (2nd ed.). Baltimore: Williams & Wilkins.

Wagner, E. H., Grothaus, L. C., Hecht, J. A., & LaCroix, A. Z. (1991). Factors associated with participation in a senior health promotion program. *Gerontologist, 31,* 598–602.

Wagner, E. H., LaCroix, A. Z., Grothaus, L., Leveille, S. G., Hecht, J. A., Artz, K., Odle, K., & Buchner, D. M. (1994). Preventing disability and falls in older adults: A population-based randomized trial. *American Journal of Public Health, 84,* 1800–1806.

Wallace, J. I., Buchner, D. M., Grothaus, L., Leveille, S., LaCroix, A. Z., & Wagner, E. H. (1998). Implementation and effectiveness of a community-based health promotion program for older adults. *Journal of Gerontology, 53A,* M301–M306.

Watkins, A. J., & Kligman, E. W. (1993). Attendance patterns of older adults in a health promotion program. *Public Health Reports, 108,* 86–90.

Weiner, D. K., Duncan, P. W., Chandler, J., & Studenski, S. A. (1992). Functional reach: A marker of physical frailty. *Journal of the American Geriatrics Society, 40,* 203–207.

2

Prevention of Disease

James T. Pacala

BACKGROUND

A system of care for older populations should seek to prevent diseases that cause the greatest mortality and morbidity. Most deaths in the geriatric population are caused by heart disease, cancer, stroke, chronic lung disease, pneumonia, and influenza (Parker, Tong, Bolden, & Wingo, 1997); most of these conditions often bring high morbidity as well. Other conditions commonly leading to morbidity (and sometimes mortality) include arthritis, hearing deficits, visual problems, diabetes, Alzheimer's disease, osteoporosis, incontinence, and falls (National Center for Health Statistics, 1990).

Prevention of these conditions can be primary, secondary, or tertiary. Primary prevention precludes diseases from occurring at all. Examples of primary prevention include chemoprophylaxis for stroke, immunoprophylaxis for pneumonia and influenza, estrogen replacement therapy for heart disease and osteoporosis, and falls prevention programs. Secondary prevention extends life or reduces morbidity through detection and treatment of diseases in their early (preclinical) or unrecognized stages. Cancer screening, bone densitometry, and identification and treatment of hearing and visual deficits are examples of secondary prevention. Tertiary prevention focuses on forestalling further consequences of clinically manifest disease. Activities such as exercise programs for persons with arthritis, diet and insulin for diabetics, and bladder training are classified as tertiary prevention.

Older populations pose special considerations for disease prevention programs. Age alters the cost-effectiveness of preventive services in two competing ways. Many diseases grow more prevalent with age, so preventive services focused on these diseases have the potential to affect more cases in older than in younger populations. Conversely, older adults have fewer remaining years of life to realize the benefits of preventive services. Mammography screening illustrates the effects of these competing forces. Both the incidence of breast cancer and the predictive value of mammography rise with age, so that screening detects more cancers in older than in younger women. Compared with a younger woman, however, an older woman from whom a preclinical breast cancer has been removed is likely to succumb sooner to another illness, lessening the potential life-extending effect of mammography.

Other age-related factors weigh on the design of preventive systems. With advancing age, some risk factors for specific diseases decline in potency even though the prevalence of those diseases increases. In these instances, risk factor reduction in older adults confers less benefit to each individual but results in greater reductions in the population's overall burden of morbidity due to the sheer number of diseased persons who are older adults. For example, elevated serum cholesterol's association with coronary heart disease (CHD) decreases with age. However, since CHD prevalence increases dramatically with age, cholesterol lowering could potentially reduce the burden of CHD in older populations as much as in younger populations (in whom the risk factor is more potent but the disease is much less common).

Professional organizations have struggled with these issues as they have attempted to formulate preventive guidelines. Two organizations, the U.S. Preventive Services Task Force (1996) and the Canadian Task Force on the Periodic Health Examination (1994), have rigorously reviewed the evidence regarding a wide range of preventive activities. Table 2.1 summarizes their recommendations for the conditions causing the most morbidity and mortality in persons age 65 and older. Health care organizations striving to prevent important diseases in older populations may wish to build systems focusing on these preventive activities, emphasizing interventions that are most cost-effective and widely recommended. For example, a prevention program for older adults would seem incomplete without influenza vaccination, which has been proven not only to halve hospitalization rates for pulmonary and cardiac conditions but also to decrease overall care costs among those immunized (Nichol, Margolis, Wuorenma, & Von Sternberg, 1994). It is even more cost-effective in high-risk older adults compared with healthy seniors (Mullooly et al., 1994).

Prevention usually requires change. Whether one is quitting smoking, receiving an immunization, or undergoing mammography, changes in the behaviors of both the patient and the health care provider are necessary. Chapter 1 discusses preventive interventions designed to forestall more general functional decline, such as diet and exercise. This chapter describes principles of behavior change, their application to model systems of disease prevention, and to the degree it is known, the effectiveness of these

TABLE 2.1   Recommendations for Primary and Secondary Prevention in Older Adults

	Endorsed By:		
	USPSTF[1] and CTFPHE[2]	Either USPSTF or CTFPHE	Neither USPSTF nor CTFPHE for ALL Older Adults, but Recommended for SELECTED Persons or by Other Professional Organization
Primary Prevention:			
Aspirin Chemoprophylaxis			✓
Blood Pressure Screening	✓		
Cholesterol Screening			✓
Obesity (height and weight)		✓	
Smoking Cessation	✓		
Diabetes Screening			✓
Influenza Immunization	✓		
Pneumonia Immunization	✓		
Hormone Replacement Therapy			✓
Secondary Prevention:			
Mammography/Clinical Breast Exam	✓[3]		
Breast Self-Exam			✓
Pap Smear	✓[4]		
Digital Rectal Exam			✓
Prostate Specific Antigen Screening			✓
Fecal Occult Blood Testing			✓
Visual Impairment Screening		✓	
Hearing Impairment Screening		✓	
Cognitive Impairment Screening			✓
Bone densitometry			✓

[1] U.S. Preventive Services Task Force.
[2] CTFPHE: Canadian Task Force on the Periodic Health Examination.
[3] Mammograms to age 70 are virtually universally recommended; many organizations, including the USPSTF, recommend that mammography should be continued in women over 70 who have a reasonable life expectancy.
[4] Most organizations recommend stopping pap smear testing at age 65 for women who have had no disease detecting on routine screening up until that age.

systems. Chapters 3 and 4 deal with tertiary preventive activities for high-risk older adults.

SYSTEMS FOR PREVENTING DISEASE

The principal components of a disease prevention system are the senior population, the primary care providers, and the health care system's organizational structure. A useful conceptual framework for preventive behaviors classifies determinants of change into predisposing, enabling, and reinforcing factors (Green, Eriksen, & Schor, 1988). Predisposing factors affect the motivation to undertake preventive activities. Enabling factors determine the maintenance of preventive behaviors in providers and consumers. Reinforcing factors serve to propagate desirable preventive behaviors, primarily through feedback to providers and patients. To enhance disease-preventing behaviors, health care systems have used a variety of strategies for modifying each of these types of factors.

Modifying Predisposing Factors

Predisposing factors that influence primary providers' practice of preventive activities include attitudes toward prevention, confidence in ability to produce change in patients, personal health behaviors, demographic characteristics, and beliefs about patients' preventive behaviors (Henry, Ogle, & Snellman, 1987; Lawrence, 1990; Maheux, Pineault, & Beland, 1987). Although predisposing factors can be difficult to change, confidence and attitudes toward prevention may improve when practitioners contribute to the design of prevention programs. Practitioners can help to identify barriers to preventive activities, design preventive protocols, and plan provider training programs for preventive practice (Ockene et al., 1996; Orlandi, 1987). Unfortunately, information regarding the effectiveness of these strategies is scarce. Older adults' beliefs, attitudes, and expectations, which are influenced by their knowledge of prevention, also are important predisposing factors (Walsh & McPhee, 1992). These factors derive from a complex array of ethnicity, life experiences, religious orientation, and social stratum, none of which are malleable.

Modifying Enabling Factors

Enabling factors include patients' and providers' knowledge of prevention and the logistics of carrying out preventive activities, which are affected by practice settings, health care organizational structures, and community environments.

Providers' knowledge about prevention can be enhanced in several ways. The traditional method of continuing medical education (CME) has produced little change in provider behaviors (Davis, Thomson, Oxman, & Haynes, 1995). More directed, practical methods of increasing knowledge have shown more promise. The combined use of opinion leaders and "academic detailing" has produced positive changes in some realms of clinical care (Lomas et al., 1991; Soumerai & Avorn, 1990). One practice intervention included a 10-minute presentation by an opinion leader and a group discussion among the practice's primary providers, who identified barriers to vaccination and designed a plan to increase immunization rates. Practices receiving the intervention increased their influenza vaccination rates from 48% to 63% within 1 year; over the same period, the vaccination rate remained stable at 46% in practices not receiving the intervention (Karuza et al., 1995).

Practice guidelines also have the potential to increase providers' knowledge and expertise, although they rarely penetrate successfully into clinical practice (Flocke, Stange, & Fedirko, 1994; Weingarten et al., 1995). In conjunction with clinical aids or the removal of practical barriers, however, they tend to be implemented more widely (Grimshaw & Russell, 1993; Lomas, Anderson, Domnick-Pierre, Vayda, Enkin, & Hannah, 1989). The use of screening flow sheets in the medical record has only a modest effect on practice, as physicians tend not to fill them out (Frame, Kowulich, & Llewellyn, 1984; Madlon-Kay, 1987). Compliance with guidelines is best facilitated by relieving primary care physicians of the responsibility for remembering to initiate periodic preventive activities. Physicians welcome computer reminders and view them as an integral component of preventive care (Knight, O'Malley, & Fletcher, 1987). A cancer prevention trial reported increases in the use of several screening tests by primary care physicians during the year after computer reminders were instituted: Stool occult blood testing increased by 46%, sigmoidoscopy by 70%, and Pap smears by 37% (McPhee, Bird, Fordham, Rodnick & Osborn, 1991). Patients with hand-held preventive checklists can also prompt their primary care physicians. In one study, older adults with prevention checklists received 53% more cancer detection services than patients without checklists (Dietrich & Duhamel, 1989).

Older adults' knowledge of prevention can be expanded through the use of pamphlets, posters, videotapes, and other educational materials distributed through the mail or at clinic visits. The provision of self-help materials and telephone counseling has been reported to induce favorable changes in smokers' preventive behaviors (Curry, McBride, Grothaus, Louie, & Wagner, 1995). Local, regional, and national programs also can enhance the population's knowledge of prevention. For example, educating the public about the dangers of hypertension has contributed to a marked decline in heart disease and stroke over the past three decades. In the future, the Internet will provide an increasing opportunity for health care organizations and communities to provide large numbers of older adults with information about disease prevention.

The effects of increased knowledge of prevention can be multiplied by improvements in the logistics of delivering preventive services in the office or clinic. Because older adults often have complex medical needs, prevention is frequently neglected in a busy practice. Tools, such as patient education guides, directories of preventive services, and written scripts for discussing complex preventive tests, relieve some of the pressure on primary providers' time (Thompson, Taplin, McAfee, Mandelson, & Smith, 1995). Another solution is to share the responsibility for disease prevention between physicians and nonphysicians. Scheduling clinic visits for preventive services with specially trained nurses has succeeded moderately in altering cardiac risk factors (Imperial Cancer Research Fund OXCHECK Study Group, 1995), in promoting healthy behavioral change (Fries, Bloch, Harrington, Richardson, & Beck, 1993; Mayer et al., 1994), and in improving cancer screening rates (Cargill, Conti, Neuhauser, & McClish, 1991). One group-model HMO instituted a program of group visits, during which older adults met monthly with their nurse and primary care physician. These sessions allocated a 15-minute period for the nurse to address health maintenance issues. In a randomized trial, the rate of pneumonia vaccinations increased 154% among participants compared with 29% in the control group; flu shots increased 9% among participants compared to an 11% decline among controls (Beck, et al., 1997).

Limits on reimbursement also present barriers to use of preventive services. Physicians, keenly aware of which preventive services are covered by Medicare, tend to underuse noncovered services (Fahs, Muller, & Schechter, 1989). In response, The Health Care Financing Administration (HCFA) conducted the Medicare Preventive Services Demonstration in five sites across the United States. Medicare coverage of preventive services resulted in modest increases in their use, probable beneficial health outcomes, and no increased overall costs (Burton, Paglia, German, Shapiro, Damiano & the Medicare Prevention Services Research Team, 1995; Burton, Steinwachs, German, Shapiro, Brant, Richards, & Clark, 1995; German et al., 1995; Lave, Ives, Traven, & Kuller, 1996).

Modifying Reinforcing Factors

Once preventive behaviors have begun, their continuation often requires reinforcement. Unfortunately, the effects of disease prevention are difficult for older adults and providers to recognize. A physician may authorize mammograms for years without detecting a single case of preclinical breast cancer. Similarly, it is difficult for clinicians to "see" the effects of influenza vaccinations.

An alternative form of reinforcement is structured performance feedback (Frame, 1992). From chart audits or utilization data, clinicians receive information about how well they perform preventive activities relative to guidelines and to their peers. Calculations of how many cases have been averted through specific preventive activities, such as flu shots, are also powerful reinforcing tools. Audit-and-feedback programs have been shown to increase screening and immunization rates among primary care physicians (McPhee, Bird, Jenkins, & Fordham, 1989; Shank, Powell, & Llewelyn, 1989).

Financial incentives may also reinforce desired behaviors. Morrow, Gooding, & Clark (1995) describe a financial incentive system in a for-profit, independent practice association (IPA) health maintenance organization. Based on record audits, this HMO paid primary care physicians for performing preventive services. Although the independent effect of the incentive program could not be discerned from other concurrent interventions, the physicians' rates of screening and immunization did increase.

INNOVATIVE DISEASE PREVENTION PROGRAMS

Successful and innovative disease prevention programs often employ many of the strategies outlined above. This section describes the operation of three innovative disease prevention programs and presents some preliminary findings about their effectiveness. The first is a comprehensive preventive system in a large health care organization; the second is a method for improving preventive practices in the primary care office, an approach that is more applicable to small health care organizations with limited resources; and the third is an approach to community-based prevention.

A Comprehensive Prevention Program—The Group Health Cooperative of Puget Sound (GHCPS)

GHCPS is a large, not-for-profit, staff-model HMO with nearly 500,000 members. Taking advantage of its centralized influence over the delivery of a broad range of health care services, GHCPS has implemented a multi-faceted disease prevention program over the past two decades (Thompson et al., 1995). The program is built on the concept of epidemiologically derived, population-based care. To initiate and guide the program, GHCPS created a committee on prevention, whose members came from multiple levels in the organization: primary care physicians and nurses at the provider level; clinic managers, researchers, quality assessors, and information system personnel at the infrastructural level; and publicists, marketers, and lobbyists at the organization and community levels. This committee regularly reviews the epidemiologic evidence regarding the effectiveness of various disease prevention activities, decides which activities to implement, and oversees development of specific programs (including guideline development).

Two preventive programs for seniors for which GHCPS has outcome data focus on breast cancer and cigarette smoking. In both programs, practitioners are involved in the identification of barriers and in the design of training curricula. The breast cancer screening program features an automated information and reminder system. Regular scans of a computer database identify women who are appropriate for screening and generate mailed reminders to them. Primary care physicians receive lists of women in their practices who are due for screening and feedback regarding their rates of adherence to the GHCPS guideline for breast cancer screening. At the community level, GHCPS has worked with several organizations to increase community awareness of the importance of breast cancer screening. Additionally, GHCPS personnel have provided testimony in Congress in support of Medicare and Medicaid coverage of screening mammography.

As a result, 65% of women have undergone mammography within 1 year of a screening invitation; nationally in 1990, less than 50% of women had undergone mammography within the previous two years (National Center for Health Statistics, 1992). At GHCPS, 84% of female enrollees older than the age of 50 have had at least one mammogram, compared to a national proportion of 67% in 1992 (Martin, Calle, Wingo, & Health, 1996). The incidence of late-stage breast cancer at diagnosis has decreased by 32% over a 5-year implementation period.

GHCPS has implemented a similar immunization program featuring a computer tracking system that provides regular information to individual practices about their patients' immunization status. GHCPS has also worked at the community level to raise awareness of influenza immunizations, and it provides free vaccine in underserved areas. Yearly influenza vaccination rates among enrollees age 65 and older rose from 34% in 1984 to 70% in 1994.

GHCPS's tobacco cessation program utilizes workshops and educational programs for physicians and patients. Patients who desire to quit receive self-help materials and telephone counseling. The GHCPS benefit package includes medical coverage for smoking cessation intervention. Over the past 11 years, referrals to this program have increased 11-fold, and use of self-help manuals has increased 20-fold. Smoking prevalence in GHCPS enrollees age 20 and over decreased from 25% to 17% from 1987 to 1994, a rate of decrease of 0.83% per year, whereas smoking prevalence in the United States over this same period decreased about 0.5% per year.

Office-Based Disease Prevention—The GAPS Approach

Dietrich, Woodruff, & Carney (1994) propose a multifaceted method for improving office-based preventive services that involves four steps: (1) setting practice goals for preventive care, (2) assessing current performance in attaining those goals, (3) planning changes in office practices to increase preventive services, and (4) starting and maintaining the interventions. This Continuous Quality Improvement (CQI)-like model allows practices to individualize their approaches to disease prevention. The GAPS (goal setting, assessment, planning, and starting) approach also stresses the importance of teamwork, with active involvement of receptionists, medical technicians, nurses, nurse practitioners, and primary care physicians in the design and implementation of preventive services.

The most important goal-setting task (Step 1) is for the practice to decide which preventive services to provide, the target population for those services, and the performance level to achieve. In Step 2, members of the health care team assess how the practice currently provides preventive services by auditing patient charts to determine performance levels. Step 3 involves designing preventive materials (e.g., patient education materials, health maintenance flow sheets, and stickers for flagging the charts of patients who have preventive needs) and altering office schedules to allow time for preventive activities (usually performed by nonphysicians). In Step 4, the office activates the program and conducts follow-up audits and staff meetings to assess how well the interventions are working. All staff members receive performance feedback.

Research on the GAPS method shows that it can be taught to and adopted by primary care practices quickly (Carney, Dietrich, Keller, Landgraf, & O'Connor; 1992). A randomized trial compared the effects of the GAPS method with a physician education approach for increasing cancer screening rates in individual primary care practices (Dietrich et al., 1992). The trial randomly assigned 98 offices to receive one, both, or neither intervention. The educational intervention consisted of a 1-day meeting in which physicians received recommendations for cancer screening. In the GAPS-like intervention, a facilitator visited the practices to provide assistance in assessing their preventive care and in designing practice-based changes to facilitate cancer screening. These changes often included practical methods for implementing health maintenance flow sheets, affixing stickers to smokers' charts, and distributing health education materials and patient health diaries.

Twelve months after the interventions, the use of cancer preventive services increased significantly more in practices receiving the GAPS-like intervention than in practices receiving the educational intervention. Practices receiving the GAPS-like intervention increased their rates of stool occult blood testing (OBT) from 48% to 62% of eligible patients; those given both interventions increased their OBT rates from 43% to 61%; those given only physician education increased their OBT rates from 48% to 54%; these given neither intervention showed virtually no change (45% to 46%).

Community-Based Prevention—The Prevention for Elderly Persons (PEP) Program

The PEP program targets its preventive effort to community sites (Reuben et al., 1996). In 1993 the UCLA Multi-campus Program in Geriatric Medicine and Gerontology formed a partnership with the Los Angeles Area Agency on Aging, a federally and locally funded service organization for older adults. The goal of the program was to identify the disease preventive needs of community-dwelling older adults and to employ effective intervention strategies to meet those needs. A four-step process lay at the program's core:

1. At community-based meal sites, nonphysicians (health educators, research associates, college students) screened seniors for preventive needs.
2. A computer program interpreted the results of the screen and produced a "prescription for prevention" that instructed and encouraged favorable behavioral change, encouraged patients to discuss specific disease preventive strategies with their physicians, and provided general information on prevention.
3. A trained health educator followed up with a telephone call to screened seniors to discuss the prescription for prevention.
4. A geriatrician telephoned screened seniors' primary physicians to discuss the recommendations generated by the health screening.

For each participant, the program required about 30 minutes to administer the screen, 20 minutes of secretarial time, 20 minutes of a master's level health educator's time, and 10 minutes of a geriatrician's time.

The first 920 participants who went through the program averaged 75 years of age, one third being from low-income households and 35% representing ethnic minorities. As yet, there are no data on the rates of subsequent preventive activities, but each participant received an average of 6.3 recommendations for discussion with their physicians. Among the most common were recommendations for aspirin prophylaxis (68%), pneumonia vaccination (61%), and colorectal cancer screening (51%). The program met several obstacles, the most formidable of which was difficulty in completing the telephone follow-up with participants and physicians. The health educator was unable to contact more than one third of the participants, and the geriatrician could not reach 35% of the patients' primary physicians.

RECOMMENDATIONS

From the evidence currently available, effective disease prevention pro-grams for older populations should include the following (see Figure 2.1):

1. *A focus on clinically important diseases for which preventive practices have been shown to be effective.* These practices include blood pressure screen-ing, smoking cessation, influenza and pneumonia immunization, mammography coupled with clinical breast exams, Pap smears, and screening for visual and hearing impairment (see Table 2.1). Screening for obesity and colon cancer probably deserve systemwide develop-ment as well. In addition, systems should screen subgroups at high risk for specific diseases, such as persons with overt coronary artery disease for hypercholesterolemia and diabetics for obesity. Programs should target particularly lower socioeconomic persons, as they tend to underuse preventive services.

2. *Knowledgeable and motivated recipients of care.* Pamphlets, posters, and self-help materials all influence older adults' knowledge of and atti-tudes toward disease prevention. Preventive counseling is most effectively and efficiently carried out telephonically or face-to-face by nonphysicians who are grounded in behavioral change theory.

3. *Practitioners' involvement in program design.* Practitioners should review new prevention literature, help to define the barriers to prac-ticing prevention, and be involved with the design of workable pre-vention programs.

4. *Knowledgeable providers.* Clear, evidence-based geriatric preventive guidelines should be readily available to providers.

5. *Practice environments that enhance preventive activities.* Telephone fol-low-up, computer reminders, and involvement of nonphysician per-sonnel enhance guideline compliance.

6. *Preventive activities in the community.* A health care organization can work with local, regional, and national agencies to promote preventive behaviors through mass mailings, public education programs, and the Internet. Organizations can also work with legislative entitles to pro-vide funding for community-based disease prevention activities.

7. *Incentives to sustain preventive behaviors.* Programs should consider providing financial incentives to practitioners for fulfilling disease prevention goals. In addition, practitioners should receive feedback on how well their practice achieved certain prevention goals. The CQI approach easily applies to preventive activities and is a good way of accomplishing favorable change and sustaining it.

As new information about the effectiveness of disease preventive activi-ties emerges, health systems will need to incorporate new strategies for

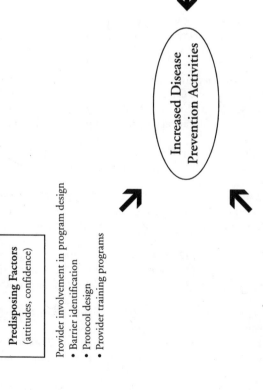

Predisposing Factors
(attitudes, confidence)

Provider involvement in program design
- Barrier identification
- Protocol design
- Provider training programs

Enabling Factors
(knowledge, logistics)

Providers
Opinion leaders/academic detailing
Practice guidelines
Computer reminders/flow sheets
Nonphysician providers
Expanded reimbursement

Patients
Patient education materials
Patient information lines/web sites
Public education through the media

Increased Disease Prevention Activities

Reinforcing Factors
(rewards)

Performance feedback
- Compliance with guidelines
- Calculated rates of diseases prevented
- Expected detection of rare events
Financial rewards

FIGURE 2.1   Evidence-based strategies for preventive activities.

encouraging its use. Effective systems of disease prevention will help older adults to remain healthy and highly functioning for as long as possible. They will also serve older adults who have already acquired chronic illnesses, the subject of the next section of this book.

REFERENCES

Beck, A., Scott, J., Williams, P., Robertson, B., Jackson, D., Gade, G., & Cowan, P. (1997). A randomized trial of group outpatient visits for chronically ill older HMO members: The Cooperative Health Care Clinic. *Journal of the American Geriatrics Society, 45*, 543–549.

Burton, L. C., Paglia, M. J., German, P. S., Shapiro, S., Damiano, A. M., & the Medicare Prevention Services Research Team. (1995). The effect among older persons of a general preventive visit on three health behaviors: Smoking, excessive alcohol drinking, and sedentary lifestyle. *Preventive Medicine, 24*, 492–497.

Burton, L. C., Steinwachs, D. M., German, P. S., Shapiro, S., Brant, L. J., Richards, T. M., & Clark, D. R. (1995). Preventive services for the elderly: Would coverage affect utilization and costs under Medicare? *American Journal of Public Health, 85*, 387–391.

Canadian Task Force on the Periodic Health Examination. (1994). *Canadian guide to clinical preventive health care.* Ottawa: Canada Communication Group.

Cargill, V. A., Conti, M., Neuhauser, D., & McClish, D. (1991). Improving the effectiveness of screening for colorectal cancer by involving nurse clinicians. *Medical Care, 29*, 1–5.

Carney, P. A., Dietrich, A. J., Keller, A., Landgraf, J., & O'Connor, G. T. (1992). Tools, teamwork, and tenacity: An office system for cancer prevention. *Journal of Family Practice, 35*, 385–387.

Curry, S. J., McBride, C., Grothaus, L. C., Louie, D., & Wagner, E. H. (1995). A randomized trial of self-help materials, personalized feedback, and telephone counseling with nonvolunteer smokers. *Journal of Consulting and Clinical Psychology, 63*, 1005–1014.

Davis, D. A., Thomson, M. A., Oxman, A. D., & Haynes, R. B. (1995). Changing physician performance: A systematic review of the effect of continuing medical education strategies. *Journal of the American Medical Association, 274*, 700–705.

Dietrich, A. J., & Duhamel, M. (1989). Improving geriatric preventive care through a patient-held checklist. *Family Medicine, 21*, 195–198.

Dietrich, A. J., O'Connor, G. T., Keller, A., Carney, P. A., Levy, D., & Whaley, F. S. (1992). Cancer: Improving early detection and prevention. A community practice randomized trial. *British Medical Journal, 304*, 687–691.

Dietrich, A. J., Woodruff, C. B., & Carney, P. A. (1994). Changing office routines to enhance preventive care: The preventive GAPS approach. *Archives of Family Medicine, 3*, 176–183.

Fahs, M. C., Muller, C., & Schechter, M. (1989). Primary medical care for elderly patients: Part 2. Results of a survey of office-based clinicians. *Journal of Community Health, 14,* 89–98.

Flocke, S. A., Stange, K. C., & Fedirko, T. L. (1994). Dissemination of information about the U.S. Preventive Services Task Force guidelines. *Archives of Family Medicine, 3,* 1006–1008.

Frame, P. S. (1992). Health maintenance in clinical practice: Strategies and barriers. *American Family Physician, 45,* 1192–1200.

Frame, P. S., Kowulich, B. A., & Llewellyn, A. M. (1984). Improving physician compliance with a health maintenance protocol. *Journal of Family Practice, 19,* 341–344.

Fries, J. F., Bloch, D. A., Harrington, H., Richardson, N., & Beck, R. (1993). Two-year results or a randomized controlled trial of a health promotion program in a retiree population: The Bank of America Study. *American Journal of Medicine, 94,* 455–462.

German, P. S., Burton, L. C., Shapiro, S., Steinwachs, D. M., Tsuji, I., Paglia, M. J., & Damiano, A. M. (1995). Extended coverage for preventive services for the elderly: Response and results in a demonstration population. *American Journal of Public Health, 85,* 379–386.

Green, L. W., Eriksen, M. P., & Schor, E. L. (1988). Preventive practices by physicians: Behavioral determinants and potential interventions. *American Journal of Preventive Medicine, 4,* S101–107.

Grimshaw, J. M., & Russell, I. T. (1993). Effect of clinical guidelines on medical practice: A systematic review of rigorous evaluations. *Lancet, 342,* 1317–1322.

Henry, R. C., Ogle, K. S., & Snellman, L. A. (1987). Preventive medicine: Physician practices, beliefs, and perceived barriers for implementation. *Family Medicine, 19,* 110–113.

Imperial Cancer Research Fund OXCHECK Study Group. (1995). Effectiveness of health checks conducted by nurses in primary care: Final results of the OXCHECK study. *British Medical Journal, 310,* 1099–1104.

Karuza, J., Calkins, E., Feather, J., Hershey, C. O., Katz, L., & Majeroni, B. (1995). Enhancing physician adoption of practice guidelines. *Archives of Internal Medicine, 155,* 625–632.

Knight, B. P., O'Malley, M. S., & Fletcher, S. W. (1987). Physician acceptance of a computerized health maintenance prompting program. *American Journal of Preventive Medicine, 3,* 19–24.

Lave, J. R., Ives, D. G., Traven, N. D., & Kuller, L. H. (1996). Evaluation of a health promotion demonstration program for the rural elderly. *HSR: Health Services Research, 31,* 261–281.

Lawrence, R. S. (1990). Diffusion of the U.S. Preventive Services Task Force recommendations into practice. *Journal of General Internal Medicine, 5,* S99–S103.

Lomas, J., Anderson, G. M., Domnick-Pierre, K., Vayda, E., Enkin, M. W., & Hannah, W. J. (1989). Do practice guidelines guide practice? The effect of a consensus statement on the practice of physicians. *New England Journal of Medicine, 321,* 1306–1311.

Lomas, J., Enkin, M., Anderson, G. M., Hannah, W. J., Vayda, E., & Singer, J. (1991). Opinion leaders vs. audit and feedback to implement practice guidelines: Delivery after previous cesarean section. *Journal of the American Medical Association, 265,* 2202–2207.

Madlon-Kay, D. J. (1987). Improving the periodic health examination: Use of a screening flow check for patients and physicians. *Journal of Family Practice, 25,* 470–473.

Maheux, B., Pineault, R., & Beland, F. (1987). Factors influencing physicians' orientation toward prevention. *American Journal of Preventive Medicine, 3,* 12–18.

Martin, L. M., Calle, E. E., Wingo, P. A., & Health, Jr., C. W. (1996). Comparison of mammography and Pap test use from the 1987 and 1992 National Health Interview Surveys: Are we closing the gaps? *American Journal of Preventive Medicine, 12,* 82–90.

Mayer, J. A., Jermanovich, A., Wright, B. L., Elder, J. P., Drew, J. A., & Williams, S. J. (1994). Changes in health behaviors of older adults: The San Diego Medicare Preventive Health Project. *Preventive Medicine, 23,* 127–133.

McPhee, S. J., Bird, J. A., Fordham, D., Rodnick, J. E., & Osborn, E. H. (1991). Promoting cancer prevention activities by primary care physicians: Results of a randomized, controlled trial. *Journal of the American Medical Association, 266,* 538–544.

McPhee, S. J., Bird, J. A., Jenkins, C. N. H., & Fordham, D. (1989). Promoting cancer screening: A randomized controlled trial of three interventions. *Archives of Internal Medicine, 149,* 1866–1872.

Morrow, R. W., Gooding, A. D., & Clark, C. (1995). Improving physicians' preventive health care behavior through peer review and financial incentives. *Archives of Family Medicine, 4,* 165–169.

Mullooly, J. P., Bennett, M. D., Hornbrook, M. C., Barker, W. H., Williams, W. W., Patriarca, P. A., & Rhodes, P. H. (1994). Influenza vaccination programs for elderly persons: Cost-effectiveness in a health maintenance organization. *Annals of Internal Medicine, 121,* 947–952.

National Center for Health Statistics. (1990). Current estimates from the National Health Interview Survey, 1989. *Vital and Health Statistics, 10,* 176.

National Center for Health Statistics. (1992). *Prevention profile: Health, United States, 1991.* Hyattsville, MD: Public Health Service.

Nichol, K. L., Margolis, K. L. Wuorenma, J., & Von Sternberg, T. (1994). The efficacy and cost effectiveness of vaccination against influenza among elderly persons living in the community. *New England Journal of Medicine, 331,* 778–784.

Ockene, I. S., Merriam, P. A., Hebert, J. R., Hurley, T. G., Ockene, J. K., & Saperia, G. M. (1996). Effect of training and a structured office practice on physician-delivered nutrition counseling: The Worcester-area trial for counseling in hyperlipidemia (WATCH). *American Journal of Preventive Medicine, 12,* 252–258.

Orlandi, M. A. (1987). Promoting health and preventing disease in health care settings: An analysis of barriers. *Preventive Medicine, 16,* 119–130.

Parker, S. L., Tong, T., Bolden, S., & Wingo, P. A. (1997). Cancer statistics, 1997. *CA–A Cancer Journal for Clinicians, 47,* 5–27.

Reuben, D. B., Hirsch, S. H., Frank, J. C., Maly, R. C., Schlesinger, M. S., Weintraub, N., & Yancey, S. (1996). The Prevention for Elderly Persons (PEP) Program: A model of municipal and academic partnership to meet the needs of older persons for preventive services. *Journal of the American Geriatrics Society, 44,* 1394–1398.

Shank, J. C., Powell, T., & Llewelyn, J. (1989). A five-year demonstration project associated with improvement in physician health maintenance behavior. *Family Medicine, 21,* 273–278.

Soumerai, S. B., & Avorn, J. (1990). Principles of educational outreach ("academic detailing") to improve clinical decision making. *Journal of the American Medical Association, 263,* 549–556.

Thompson, R. S., Taplin, S. H., McAfee, T. A., Mandelson, M. T., & Smith, A. E. (1995). Primary and secondary prevention services in clinical practice: Twenty years' experience in development, implementation, and evaluation. *Journal of the American Medical Association, 273,* 1130–1135.

U.S. Preventive Services Task Force. (1996). Guide to clinical preventive services (2nd ed.). Baltimore: Williams & Wilkins.

Walsh, J. M. E., & McPhee, S. J. (1992). A systems model of clinical preventive care: An analysis of factors influencing patient and physician. *Health Education Quarterly, 19,* 157–175.

Weingarten, S., Stone, E., Hayward, R., Tunis, S., Pelter, M., Huang, H., & Kristopaitis, R. (1995). The adoption of preventive care practice guidelines by primary care physicians: Do actions match intentions? *Journal of General Internal Medicine, 10,* 138–144.

II

When the Older Person Is Chronically Ill or at Risk

*S*ixty percent of people over the age of 64 years have two or more chronic illnesses. Within this chronically ill population is a small group (10% of the whole older population) whose conditions are unstable and prone to exacerbation. Its members suffer frequent health-related crises that consume about 70% of all resources used by older persons.

The needs of these chronically ill seniors are multifaceted and complex, psychological and social, as well as medical. The care they need is complicated, often requiring several facilities, providers from different disciplines, and payment from multiple sources. The results are predictable: disorganization, inefficiency, high cost, suboptimal health, and low levels of satisfaction (among patients, families, providers, and purchasers).

Recently, increasing effort has been expended to create order from this chaos. Chronically ill older persons are being regarded as challenging rather than hopeless, deserving of comprehensive evaluation and coordinated proactive interdisciplinary care. They and their families are being encouraged to be active participants. Even more recently, rigorous studies of the clinical and financial outcomes of novel applications of these principles have been launched. The following two chapters describe several innovative programs (now under evaluation) that are designed to

- *enhance the effectiveness of the primary care of older persons with chronic conditions*
- *identify and proactively treat seniors who are at high risk for adverse outcomes in the future*

3

Care of Older People With Chronic Illness

Edward H. Wagner

Chronic illness is an important aspect of aging. Nearly three quarters of adults 65 years and older report one or more chronic illness, and nearly half report two or more. For example, fully one quarter of all seniors report the cooccurence of hypertension and arthritis. Chronic illness significantly diminishes one's current health and functional status and increases the risk of future disability and mortality. Kosorok examined the relationships among restricted activity days (an important measure of dysfunction), age, gender, and the presence or absence of various health conditions in the Supplement on Aging to the 1984 National Health Interview Survey (Kosorok, Omenn, Diehr, Koepsell, Patrick, 1992). The average noninstitutionalized American age 65 or older restricted his or her usual activities because of illness or injury on 31 days a year. In multivariate analyses, it was the presence of health conditions, not age, that accounted for increases in restricted activity days. Chronic diseases like arthritis, heart disease, and hypertension accounted for 18 of the 31 days, with falls, a common complication of chronic disease in the elderly, accounting for another 6 days.

In another survey, older persons were asked to report difficulties performing tasks and to indicate the cause of these difficulties. Most attributed them to chronic illness, most often to arthritis (49%) or heart disease (14%) (Ettinger, Fried, Harris, Shemanski, & Shultz, for the CHS Collaborative Research Group, 1994). Only 12% attributed their dysfunction to old age.

In contrast to the clear cross-sectional association between chronic illness and the inability to function normally, the evidence that specific chronic illnesses predict future dysfunction is more mixed. Cohort studies show that stroke and dementia consistently predict future dysfunction, that arthritis and depressive symptoms predict dysfunction in most stud-ies, but that heart disease, diabetes, and hypertension are inconsistent predictors. Guralnick found that prevalent, but not incident, diabetes was predictive of mobility loss (Guralnick et al., 1993). Since the complications of diabetes and other chronic illnesses are strongly related to the duration of disease, the inclusion of recent cases may help explain prior inconsis-tencies in earlier studies. Long-standing chronic illnesses are also associ-ated with a greater prevalence of co-morbid conditions, and combinations of chronic illness may increase the extent of subsequent disability.

THE ETIOLOGY OF DISABILITY IN CHRONIC ILLNESS

The links between chronic disease and disability result from the direct effects of the illness on physiologic reserve either through tissue damage (e.g., stroke limiting mobility, or cataract limiting vision) or through dis-comfort (e.g., osteoarthritic pain limiting lower extremity function). Chronic illness also affects function indirectly through deconditioning and depression. Deconditioning can be acute, as seen in hospitalized older patients (Bortz, 1982), or slowly progressive as a result of declines in phys-ical activity associated with the longer-term effects of chronic disease or the effects of treatment. Ill health also appears to be a major reason for dropouts from exercise programs (Kriska et al., 1986).

Another link between chronic disease and deconditioning may relate to the observation that older people are more cautious than their younger counterparts and may be more likely to reduce activities for fear of exac-erbating their chronic illness. For example, fear of falling has been associ-ated with declines in health and increases in health care utilization (Maki, Holliday, & Topper, 1991). Older persons with chronic illnesses thus have multiple reasons for becoming deconditioned, a fact that must be addressed in efforts to improve outcomes (Wagner, LaCroix, Buchner, & Larson, 1992).

The relationships among chronic disease, depression, and disability are being clarified by longitudinal study. Approximately 20% of all individ-uals 65 years or older report substantial symptoms of depression—sad-ness, fatigue, withdrawal, insomnia. Depression is clearly associated with reduced activity and may contribute to noncompliance with medication. Regardless of whether depression predisposes to chronic disease or vice versa, depressive diagnoses or symptoms independently predict future dysfunction (Bruce, Seeman, Merrill, & Blazer, 1994). The detection and effective management of depression must be a consideration for any sys-tematic effort to improve outcomes in chronic illness.

THE "NATURAL HISTORY" OF CHRONIC DISEASE

Most chronic illnesses wax and wane for the remainder of the older person's life, although these fluctuations occur around a generally downward trajectory. Exacerbations contribute in a major way to the pathophysiologic damage, deconditioning, and depression that determine the disability associated with chronic illnesses (Buchner & Wagner, 1992). Many seniors experiencing acute illness or injury fail to recover completely to pre-exacerbation levels. Obviously, the more frequent and severe the exacerbations and the longer the periods of deconditioning, the less likely will be full recovery. If this postulated natural history is correct, then management of chronic illness must be directed to the prevention of exacerbations and complications and to the prevention of functional loss during exacerbations.

As discussed in earlier chapters, epidemiologic studies and intervention trials have repeatedly shown that older people, even those with chronic conditions, can improve their health status and function. A significant percentage (usually 15% to 20%) of individuals with ADL limitations will regain their function in a year or more. For example, we have found that 18% of chronically ill seniors who received disability prevention and chronic disease self-management support interventions demonstrated better performance of activities of daily living than they did 1 year earlier (Leveille et al., 1998). Thus, even those seniors with established chronic illness do not face relentless decline.

THERAPY FOR CHRONIC ILLNESS

Through advances in therapy, considerable progress has been made in reducing the fatal and morbid consequences of diseases like hypertension, arteriosclerotic cardiovascular and cerebrovascular disease, congestive heart failure, and atrial fibrillation. As a result of these advances, the outcomes of chronic illness increasingly depend upon the appropriate application of state-of-the-art therapy. For example, coronary heart disease mortality was reduced among Medicare beneficiaries with acute myocardial infarction who received aspirin as compared to those who didn't (Krumholtz et al., 1996). The list of those treatments proven by randomized trials to improve outcomes gets longer by the year: angiotensin converting enzyme (ACE) inhibitors for congestive heart failure and diabetic nephropathy, low-dose diuretics for systolic hypertension, warfarin for atrial fibrillation, hormones and alendronate for osteoporosis, and organized foot care and education for patients with diabetes.

These proven treatments include educational and supportive interventions as well as drugs and surgical procedures. Behavior changes are critical elements in the successful management of many chronic conditions. Optimal treatment often necessitates increasing physical activity, strengthening peripheral and pelvic musculature, eliminating cigarette smoking, inspecting feet, taking medication correctly, modifying diet, and other behavioral changes.

Effective therapies also minimize those chronic symptoms that interfere with function or other elements of treatment. These include pharmacotherapy to control symptoms of conditions like arthritis, chronic obstructive pulmonary disease (COPD), Parkinson's disease, incontinence, and benign prostatic hyperplasia, as well as behaviors like Kegel exercises to reduce symptoms of incontinence and dietary modification to relieve the discomfort of constipation and gastroesophageal reflux.

The growing list of effective interventions presents challenges to practices and health care systems to ensure their consistent delivery to all relevant patients. The effective delivery of some of the interventions requires skills and resources often not found in usual medical practice—scientific behavior change counseling, functional assessment methods, proactive follow-up. Therefore, programs and approaches to improve outcomes in chronic illness must make certain that these skills are accessible to each practice and that systems are in place to ensure their consistent delivery to older persons.

THE PATIENT'S ROLE IN EFFECTIVE CHRONIC ILLNESS MANAGEMENT

The primary providers of chronic illness care are, of course, patients and their nonprofessional caregivers. State-of-the-art therapy is useless if unused or contravened by dietary or other behavioral indiscretions, or if ominous symptoms are disregarded. Self-management, which is among the central tasks confronting patients as they negotiate their illnesses, includes self-monitoring, changing lifestyle, dealing with the emotional impacts, and interacting with the health care system (Clark et al., 1991). Medical care can either assist and support patients and caregivers in meeting their self-management responsibilities or undermine them, leading to passivity and dependency. The ability of patients to manage their illnesses is enhanced by relationships with a provider team capable of sharing decision-making and treatment planning and by involvement in activities and programs designed to increase confidence and skills in self-management (Von Korff, Gruman, Schaefer, Curry, & Wagner, 1997). These issues will be explored in more depth later in this chapter and in chapter 17.

CURRENT PRACTICE

By most available measures, the usual care of older persons with chronic illness fails to meet evidence-based guidelines and the needs of patients. Survey after survey, audit after audit have demonstrated that sizable percentages of patients with diseases like diabetes, congestive heart failure, hypertension, coronary heart disease, and atrial fibrillation are not receiving treatments proven to be effective (Wagner, Austin, & Von Korff, 1996b). Although much more difficult to study, patient education, behavioral interventions, and psychosocial support appear to be even less likely to be delivered in a consistent, state-of-the-art manner.

Barriers to Effective Chronic Illness Management

To improve outcomes in chronic illness, health systems must ensure that

1. exacerbations are identified early in their course and treated appropriately
2. patients are making behavioral adjustments to control the illness and prevent deconditioning
3. effective therapy is prescribed and taken
4. patients are given support and resources to help them manage the emotional and social impacts of the illness

To meet these objectives routinely for the several hundred older persons in the typical generalist's practice is extremely difficult for even the most conscientious and highly trained provider. The problem is that the usual generalist practice is oriented to providing acute care for urgent problems (Kottke, Brekke, & Solberg, 1993; Wagner, Austin, & VonKorff, 1996a).

Characteristics reflective of this orientation include the reliance on patient-initiated interactions, the predominance of the 15-minute (or shorter) office visit, the emphasis on symptoms rather than function or quality of life, and the rarity of organized systems of patient education and follow-up. Hirsch and Winograd (1996) studied geriatric care in California primary care practices and found that few routinely scheduled longer visits for older patients or had standard approaches for the assessment of function. Rushed visits initiated by patients to address their symptoms make it very difficult to accomplish the tasks needed for effective chronic illness care and often lead to additions to an already complicated drug regimen. It is not for lack of contact that effective care is not provided; chronically ill seniors see their physicians every month or two on average. The visits are often not productive.

Medical Care for Patients With Chronic Illness

Whether part of an organized program or not, care for seniors with chronic illness most often revolves around a single primary professional caregiver (see Figure 3.1). The primary caregiver, in most cases is a generalist physician and is part of a practice team, which, depending on its composition, supports the physician and delivers additional services. In most practices, the team includes nurses and, to a more variable extent, pharmacists and social workers. The practice team works within a health care system that may be no larger than the team itself, or it may be a complex and byzantine corporate giant. That system provides the supports for the work of the practice team—space, medical records, clinical policies, computers, and access to other professionals. This simple depiction of a practice as a "target" affords a convenient way of describing and categorizing interventions designed to improve outcomes in older adults with chronic illness. Interventions may aim to influence primary caregivers, the practice team, or the system in attempting to improve chronic illness care.

Successful interventions for improving outcomes for chronically ill seniors usually use one of two quite distinctive strategies: They either enhance the work of the usual practice team or they bypass it by creating a new care-giver and team. The former, while more acceptable to primary care–based systems, is more difficult to implement and has not been well studied with multiproblem, frail seniors. Some approaches appear to fall in the middle in the sense that they create a new team whose role is to enhance the care of the usual team. Such hybrid programs (e.g., outpatient geriatric consultation services) can be categorized as either enhancing or bypassing by the extent to which they assume management of the patients' problems.

Two factors seem to influence the selection of the strategy: the nature of the larger system and the complexity and severity of the illness. Most commercial "disease management" programs favor the bypass strategy, probably because their major clients are independent practice associations (IPAs) or network model health plans with relatively few enrollees in each of many practices, or self-insurance groups that are trying to reduce costs. Group/staff model HMOs, with stronger links to practices, tend to favor the enhancement model. Strategies to improve care for more common and less complex conditions such as hypertension or osteoarthritis tend to favor enhancement approaches, whereas bypass approaches are favored for more complex and severe conditions like HIV/AIDS and Alzheimer's disease.

The Primary Professional Caregiver

In usual medical care, the identification of the primary professional caregiver is unambiguous, although it can become confusing when multiple consulting specialists are involved. Interventions to improve chronic illness

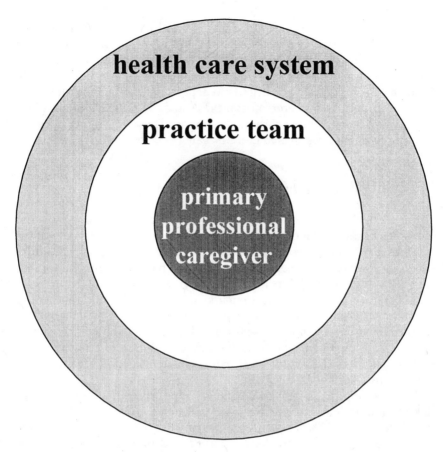

FIGURE 3.1 Organization of medical care for chronic illness.

care, however, may obscure the identification of the primary caregiver, whether of the bypass or enhancement variety. Bypass programs refer or direct patients to specialized caregivers, often nonphysician case managers, whose role in the care of the full spectrum of a patient's clinical and psychosocial needs should be carefully discussed with the primary care team. Experience suggests that these discussions often don't occur. Similarly, enhancement programs often append specialized resources such as a clinical nurse specialist or clinical pharmacist to the primary practice team. Experience suggests that in some practices these new personnel function as consultants and supports; more often they begin to assume the role of primary professional caregiver.

Thus many of the early efforts to improve the quality and/or reduce the costs of chronic illness care have transgressed cherished values in

Western medicine—the primacy of the personal physician, continuity of care, and comprehensiveness of services. In the future, will new modes of sharing care among generalist and specialized providers and teams improve overall outcomes, not just disease indicators, and be acceptable to older persons, or will it contribute to depersonalization, breakdowns in communication, and poorer outcomes? And how will this affect older adults, with their multiple chronic conditions? These are among the most pressing research questions in geriatric care (Wagner, 1997).

EFFECTIVE CARE FOR CHRONIC ILLNESS

The available evidence across a range of chronic conditions suggests that outcomes in chronic illness will be improved through the early identification and treatment of exacerbations and complications, appropriate application of proven treatments, and effective patient self-management. Achieving these critical functions routinely requires productive interactions between practice teams prepared to manage chronic illness and informed, activated patients (see Figure 3.2). Productive interactions are characterized by systematic assessment of functional and clinical status, collaborative treatment planning, the implementation of effective treatments, support of the patient's self-management tasks, and organized follow-up (Von Korff et al., 1997).

There is empiric as well as theoretical support for the importance of these activities. For example, Rich and colleagues (Rich et al., 1993) estimated that nearly 50% of hospitalizations of older patients with congestive heart failure were preventable. They attributed preventable hospitalizations to inadequate discharge planning, loss to follow-up, noncompliance with medications or diet, and failure to seek treatment for symptom recurrence. They then designed and tested a program to address these deficiencies through protocol-driven care management by a specially trained nurse supported by a geriatric cardiologist and other disciplines (Rich et al., 1995). With the help of a clear treatment protocol, regular contact (in-person and telephone), and standardized patient education interventions, the nurse tried to assure early detection of deterioration through symptom and weight monitoring, effective drug management, and adherence to diet and drugs. The program was evaluated through a randomized, controlled clinical trial, which showed that in comparison with usual care, the intervention reduced rehospitalizations by 56% and improved quality of life.

Assessment

The effective management of chronic illness requires the systematic collection of information about the patient's health, attitudes, behaviors, and

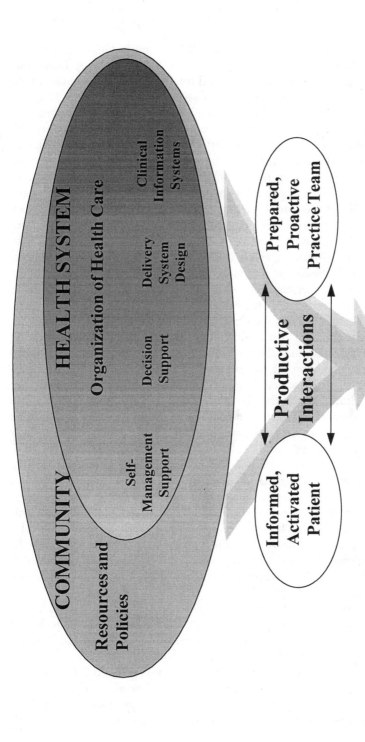

FIGURE 3.2   Chronic care improvement model.

preferences. This assessment includes the patient's view or model of the illness (Greenfield, Kaplan, Ware, Yano, & Frank, 1988; Hampson, Glasgow, & Toobert, 1990), function and quality of life, emotional adjustment to the illness (Moore & Siu, 1996), self-management behaviors, and the effectiveness of clinical and self-management. A shared understanding of the causes, natural history, and treatment of the illness (model of illness) appears to be necessary for effective management to occur. For instance, Hampson and colleagues (Hampson et al., 1990) have developed an instrument that assesses the model of illness held by patients with diabetes. Older persons and providers need not agree about all aspects of the illness (e.g., about the complementary role of alternative treatments), but agreement about the primary goals of treatment and the major intervention strategies seems critical. Since providers seldom ask older persons for their views on their illness, active intervention with patients or providers may be necessary to ensure that such discussions occur (Greenfield et al., 1988). A shared understanding is especially crucial when treatment is preventive (i.e., the effects are invisible) and involves trade-offs (e.g., improved glycemic control vs. weight gain in diabetes).

Assessment protocols for frail seniors can vary from a brief screening costing a few dollars to elaborate, multihour batteries of questionnaires and testing. In choosing the components of an assessment—whether self-reported data, performance tests, or laboratory procedures—measures should be included only if they have demonstrated reliability, validity, and responsiveness, and if they provide data necessary for treatment planning.

A standardized, office-based assessment of each patient's health, knowledge of preventive needs, and evaluation of medical care is at the heart of the Dartmouth COOP's systematic approach to improving geriatric care within its network of primary care practices (Wasson, Jette, Johnson, Mohr, & Nelson, 1997). In this model, the questionnaire is distributed to each visiting patient by office staff, and the data are put into electronic form by a bar-code reader. Software then immediately generates individualized self-care information for the patient and a flow sheet for the physician, identifying clinical and psychosocial issues needing attention. The immediacy of the information and its real-time linkage with care make this and related approaches potentially very effective.

The utility of a brief, standardized assessment is also illustrated by the work of Montgomery, Lieberman, Singh, and Fries (1994), who tested the efficacy of a patient education intervention for patients with Parkinson's disease. Their approach differed importantly from usual patient education programs in that the educational messages and recommendations were individualized on the basis of regularly collected patient data. Recipients of the intervention received mailed questionnaires every 2 months. The questionnaire contained scales assessing activities of daily living, symptoms at various times of the day, medication regimen, and number of physician visits and hospitalizations. From these data, the computer generated personalized recommendations and progress reports. These were sent in conjunction with pamphlets and other educational materials; reports of clinical status and recommendations were also sent to the patients' physicians. Two hundred ninety patients were randomly divided into intervention and control groups and were assessed at baseline and 6 months later. The intervention group patients reported significantly fewer symptoms, better quality of life, greater exercise levels, and reduced medication requirements.

Treatment Planning

The management of chronic illness confronts both patients and providers with a variety of tasks, many of which must be done repetitively at varying intervals. A senior with uncomplicated systolic hypertension and her practice team must deal with medication adjustment, dietary change, blood pressure monitoring, maintenance of a safe serum potassium level, assessment for vascular risk factors and complications, and the psychological challenges of fluctuating blood pressure levels and the increased risk of stroke and heart attack. It is essential that patient and practice agree on and understand the array of tasks and schedules required for even a comparatively straightforward illness like hypertension.

Critical pathways, which play an increasing role in acute hospital care (see chapter 7), illustrate elements of an effective treatment plan—a schedule of tasks and a clear definition of roles. But critical pathways are designed by health professionals to guide the behavior of health professionals over short periods of time (often limited to the duration of hospitalization). Effective treatment plans for chronic illnesses should guide the behaviors of both patients and professionals over long periods of time, with most of the planned activity occurring outside the medical care setting. For this reason, patients must be active participants in the development of a treatment plan since its successful execution depends heavily on their actions. The computerization of treatment plans allows elements to be updated automatically. When placed in the hands of patients, treatment plans appear to have greater potency in increasing adherence to the therapeutic regimen.

Treatment planning played a central role in a senior center–based program for chronically ill seniors conducted by our group (Leveille, Wagner, Davis, et al., 1998). Chronically ill seniors age 70 and older who were in a managed care organization and referred by their primary care physicians were enrolled in a randomized trial. The 101 patients randomized to the intervention group met with a geriatric nurse practitioner (GNP) who reviewed with the patients information from their primary care physician and from a baseline assessment of their health, functional status, health behaviors, and physical performance. The GNP and patient then developed a health action plan based on the patient's needs and priorities and a schedule for monitoring progress. The plan addressed disability risk factors, such as inactivity or depression, and the improvement of the patient's self-management skills through use of interventions made available in the senior center—for example, a self-management course (Lorig et al., 1994), a supervised exercise program (Wallace et al., 1998), and a grieving support group. The GNP regularly monitored the plan principally by telephone. When the intervention and control subjects were assessed again 6 and 12 months after randomization, the intervention subjects showed significantly less decline in function, as measured by ADLs and restricted activity days, and significantly fewer hospitalizations than controls.

Evidence-Based Clinical Management

Improving outcomes in chronically ill older adults also requires that physicians prescribe and patients take those treatments shown to be effective in improving outcomes. As will be discussed more fully below, prescription of effective therapy and other provider behaviors are complex actions influenced by a host of factors besides training and motivation (Eisenberg, 1995). The training of physicians in the theory and methods of evidence-based medicine is increasing, and more and more health systems are establishing training programs to ensure that their practitioners can evaluate the medical literature and distinguish scientifically grounded guidelines and clinical policies from anecdote and opinion. This should increase knowledge of effective therapies. Sadly, however, effective treatments aren't always administered by health professionals who know that they are effective and know how to administer them. The most cogent explanations for this disturbing fact are lack of opportunity, distraction by more visible concerns, and lack of confidence in the patient's ability to understand and adhere to the therapy. For example, depression is a major cause of morbidity and dysfunction, effective treatments are available, and yet many patients remain undetected and untreated (Wells, Katon, Rogers, & Camp 1994).

Increasing the effectiveness of clinical management in busy practices requires systematic, supportive interventions; lectures and seminars are not enough. Katon and colleagues (Katon et al., 1995) tested a multifaceted intervention to increase compliance with national guidelines for the recognition and treatment of depression. The intervention included patient education, primary care physician education, and a restructuring of appointments so that depressed patients had a longer initial visit with their primary care physician (30 vs. the usual 15 minutes). After the initial visit, the patients had four weekly visits alternating between their primary care physician and a study psychiatrist. The psychiatrist monitored pharmacy data to ensure medication compliance, while general follow-up was provided by the primary care physician. Patients randomized to the intervention arm were significantly more likely to take adequate doses of recommended medications (76% vs. 50%), and substantially more intervention patients with major depression improved clinically (74% vs. 44%).

Support for Patient Self-Management

The successful management of chronic illness depends heavily on the patient's ability to deal effectively with the self-management challenges presented by the illness and its treatment (Clark et al., 1991; Von Korff et al., 1997). There is now strong evidence that educational and supportive interventions directed to making patients better self-managers improves outcomes across a range of chronic illnesses (Von Korff et al., 1997). Effective interventions have been delivered to individuals, in groups, by telephone, and via computer. The mode of delivery may be less important to the success of a program than its content and consistency with behavioral principles. Effective interventions tend to

1. emphasize the acquisition of skills rather than just knowledge
2. systematically try to bolster patient motivation and self-efficacy rather than encourage dependency
3. pay attention to the influence of family, job, and other social influences
4. promote self-monitoring

Two highly successful self-management programs for different chronic conditions employing very different delivery approaches highlight these commonalities.

Lorig and Holman (1993) have developed and tested the cost-effectiveness of lay-led self-management groups for arthritis patients. The structured curriculum, delivered in six 2-hour sessions, is designed to increase the participants' confidence (self-efficacy) in their ability to manage the illness and to participate in decisions concerning their health care. The course also emphasizes the acquisition of specific self-management skills, such as symptom monitoring and exercise. In a series of randomized trials, arthritis patients participating in the self-management course demonstrated significantly greater knowledge of the disease and reported enhanced self-efficacy and less pain. Intervention subjects visited their physicians 40% less often, leading to cost savings as a result of the program. Although disseminated internationally by the American Rheumatism Association, remarkably few organized health systems have integrated the program into their systems.

Litzelman and colleagues (Litzelman, Slemenda, Langefield, Hays, Welch, Bild, Ford, & Vinicor, 1993) attempted to reduce diabetic foot lesions by increasing the self-management skills and confidence of patients with diabetes. They randomized low-income diabetic patients to usual care or a multifaceted intervention to prevent amputations. The core of the intervention was a series of educational sessions for one to four patients with a nurse clinician in order to observe baseline foot care, provide education through videos and pamphlets on appropriate behaviors and footwear, and negotiate a behavioral contract with each patient. The behavioral contract was reinforced by follow-up telephone calls and postcards during the following 3 months. To prompt appropriate provider behaviors, special folders, decals, and flow sheets were placed in the patients' charts. One year later, the investigators found that intervention patients were significantly more likely to be engaging in desired foot behaviors, had less than half as many serious foot lesions and significantly fewer foot infections, and were more than twice as likely to have had their feet inspected by their physicians. This study demonstrates the importance of enhancing behavioral or clinical interventions with regular follow-up and changes in office systems, the subjects of the remainder of the chapter.

Although these two programs differ in several respects, they share the features that appear to be material to the success of self-management interventions—skills training, confidence building, and sustained follow-up. In addition, they trained and encouraged patients to become more active participants in their care both at home and in the physician's office. Some programs (Anderson et al., 1995; Greenfield et al., 1988) have made patient activation or empowerment a primary goal of the intervention and have achieved improvements in attitudes, behaviors, and physiologic indicators. Patient activation interventions may be a critical element in chronic illness care and are discussed in more detail in chapter 17.

Sustained Follow-up

All of the successful chronic disease interventions described above maintained ongoing contact with their patients. In contrast with much of usual medical care, particularly in managed care settings, the practice, not the patient, bore the responsibility for initiating and sustaining follow-up. Many medical practices, unlike their dental or veterinary counterparts, have not yet developed systems for contacting patients by telephone or mail, which seriously limits the potency of their care and the ability to achieve high rates of adherence to their recommendations. High-quality care for chronic illness should follow the general methods of population-based care (Greenlick, 1992; Wagner, 1995), that is, the systematic delivery of effective interventions to all relevant members of the in-practice population. The principles of population-based care oblige practices to identify patients who need services and then act to ensure that those services are delivered.

Proactive follow-up appears to be a powerful intervention regardless of the content or approach. For example, Maisiak and colleagues (Maisiak, Austin, & Heck, 1996) studied two very different strategies for the telephone follow-up of patients with osteoarthritis (OA) and rheumatoid arthritis (RA). The first strategy, symptom monitoring, consisted simply of the repeated administration of symptom and health status questionnaires by college students, who provided no advice of any sort. The second strategy, treatment counseling, was far more interactive; it involved a review of patient self-management behaviors and then active counseling on difficulties encountered. Counselors were experienced master's level therapists. Patients in both groups were called 11 times over a 9-month interval. The results, although somewhat different for RA and OA, generally showed that, in comparison with a nonintervention control group, treatment counseling significantly improved symptoms and health status. Symptom monitoring, despite its passive nature and lack of any overtly therapeutic content, showed effects intermediate between treatment counseling and control; these differences reached statistical significance for some measures. The often expressed fear that this sort of patient contact would generate doctor visits was not confirmed by these data. OA patients in the two intervention groups actually had fewer visits than the control group, reaching statistical significance for treatment counseling.

The study described above is but one of many randomized trials that have demonstrated the powerful impact of regular practice- or system-initiated follow-up (Wasson Sanvigne Mogielnicki, Frey Soz Aandette & Rockwell 1984; Von Korff et al., 1997). These contacts afford patients opportunities to ask questions, provide information, express concerns, and receive reassurance and support. Providers receive critical information about regimen adherence, side effects, symptoms, function, and psychological status. Based on this exchange, the patient and the provider can adjust the treatment plan.

PRACTICE AND SYSTEM SUPPORTS FOR EFFECTIVE CHRONIC ILLNESS CARE

Most of the successful interventions described above did more than simply add a new intervention to practice as usual. Successful chronic disease interventions tend to be multifactorial, with components directed to the patient, to the provider(s), and to the system. As illustrated in Figure 3.2, effective chronic illness care requires a prepared provider team that can engage productively with an activated, informed patient. Preparation means having the necessary expertise to manage the illness, timely access to key clinical data, adequate time to communicate with the patient, reminders and other tools to ensure effective clinical management, and high-quality educational and consultative resources.

This stands in stark contrast to the usually rushed encounter with a near-naked older person perched uncomfortably on a cold examining table. We have reviewed the literature on the management of chronic illness in an effort to identify not only the interventions that work but also the changes in the system and practice environment that support high-quality chronic illness care (Wagner, 1996; Wagner et al., 1996a). In most instances, significant changes and enhancements to the larger practice system were necessary to support more specific intervention components such as guideline implementation, patient education, and follow-up. The common elements of these system changes fall into four general areas:

1. *Clinical information systems*—patient data that facilitate patient identification, care planning, reminders, and feedback
2. *Self-management interventions*—resources and programs to meet the information, behavior change, and psychosocial needs of patients
3. *Delivery system design*—reorganization of practice roles and office systems to support effective clinical management and follow-up
4. *Decision support*—ensuring that providers have the necessary expertise

One and usually more of these elements were found in most successful interventions. The diabetes foot care intervention discussed above (Litzelman et al., 1993) illustrates how these four elements interact to contribute to effective interventions

1. *Information systems.* All relevant diabetic patients in the practice population and their next appointment date were identified from a comprehensive computerized database. To remind providers of foot care needs, several modifications of the written medical record were generated, including a special folder, decals, and a flow sheet.
2. *Self-management interventions.* Patient education sessions relied on commercially available written and videotape resources.
3. *Delivery system design.* The intervention depended on the addition of trained nurse clinicians to the usual primary care team. Also, a follow-up system involving telephone calls and postcards was implemented.
4. *Decision support.* Flow sheets incorporating foot care practice guidelines were attached to the medical record on every visit.

In our literature review, we found that these system enhancements under-girded effective interventions across a variety of conditions, suggesting that generic approaches to chronic illness management may well meet the needs of patients with different conditions and different clinical requirements.

Information Systems

A registry, or list of all patients with a condition, is an essential first step in assisting practices in making the transition from acute, reactive care to planned, population-based interventions for older persons with chronic illness. Without it, practices must depend on patients or memory. Registries have a long history, and their advantages were recognized long before computers entered medical practice (Fry, 1973). A defined practice popu-lation, such as the enrollees of a prepaid health plan, and computerized clinical data greatly increase the feasibility of registries. A registry or a more comprehensive clinical computing system can remind patients and physicians of needed care processes (Johnston, Langton, Haynes, & Mathieu, 1994). Few interventions have more consistently increased com-pliance with practice guidelines than computerized reminders. If the reg-istry is connected to mailing lists or telephone directories, it can assist in reminding patients of needed services and scheduling them. Registries also provide feedback to providers about their performance, and they assist in treatment planning by furnishing lists of required interventions and schedules.

Self-Management Interventions

Supporting patients and families as they struggle to cope with their chron-ic illness(es) requires skilled providers, appropriate content, and effective delivery vehicles. Health systems wanting to improve their chronic illness care must ensure that all three are in place. Even though the disease and the delivery vehicle may differ (e.g., individual counseling, group ses-sions, and computer-directed), successful self-management programs are based on a collaborative process between patients and providers that defines problems, sets priorities, establishes goals, and creates treatment plans. The provider responsible for working with the patient on self-management must have the time and training to do so. Many of the successful programs in the literature have delegated this responsibility to nurses with extra experience or training in the condition of interest. The congestive heart failure intervention of Rich and colleagues described above (Rich et al., 1995) depended on an experienced cardiovascular research nurse, who provided the educational core of the intervention. Nurses with clinical training would appear to be among the most appropriate providers of self-management support, as they have training in behavioral and counseling techniques and they possess the clinical knowledge to coordinate the self-management and clinical plans and to answer patient questions and concerns.

The provider working collaboratively with the patient on self-management priorities and plans should have ready access to a range of proven self-management training and support services—classes, booklets, and videos. Effectiveness will be limited if providers have to search for educational, behavior change, or psychosocial interventions or force patients to fend for themselves. To assist providers, we have completed a review of over 400 meta-analyses and randomized trials of self-management support interventions in chronic illness (Center for the Advancement of Health, 1996). Overall, the literature indicates that there are many successful models, especially those giving emphasis to building confidence and skills rather than to imparting knowledge.

Two randomized trials of disability and fall prevention interventions for ambulatory seniors conducted by our group (Wagner et al., 1994; Wallace et al., 1998) illustrate the differential value of specific self-management resources. Both interventions involved an assessment followed by the establishment of a disability/fall prevention plan with a nurse. The follow-up interventions in the two trials differed little except for the exercise component. In the first trial, sedentary subjects were invited to attend a 2-hour exercise orientation and encouraged either to exercise on their own or to select from a list of community physical activity programs (Wagner et al., 1994). In the latter trial, all subjects were referred to a specific thrice-weekly supervised exercise program at their local senior center (Wallace et al., 1998). While intervention subjects in the earlier trial increased their exercise minimally and showed only modest health improvements compared to controls, nearly all subjects in the latter trial participated actively in the exercise program and substantially improved their physical performance and health status compared to controls.

Health systems should identify a small set of effective self-management materials and programs and ensure that both providers and patients know how to access it. For older persons, many of these self-management support resources will reside outside the health care delivery system in senior centers, community agencies, volunteer organizations, and home nursing services. Expanding and strengthening the links between health care organizations and community resources would appear to be a high priority for those organizations wanting to improve care for its older enrollees. These links can be at the institutional level, through contracted services or jointly funded activities, or at the practice level. An example of the latter is the work of Wendy Levinson and colleagues in Portland, Oregon, testing the effectiveness of adding a resource specialist to the practice team. The role of the resource specialist is to identify needs for community services among seniors in the practice and to assist them in finding the most appropriate resources. Typical resources sought include safe and effective exercise options, nutritional counseling and meal support, transportation, and adaptive equipment.

Delivery System Design

Successful chronic illness initiatives, in contrast to usual primary medical care, design or change their delivery systems to meet the needs of patients with chronic illnesses. Escaping the constraints of reactive busy practice requires significant effort. For most systems, this includes changes in provider relationships, practice team organization and task delegation, appointment and follow-up systems, and the availability of key specialty resources. The most critical design decision is the determination of where responsibility for care of the chronically ill senior resides. Does accountability remain with the primary care provider and team, or is it transferred in whole or in part to a "case manager" or specialized geriatric care team? Most successful programs in the literature either conduct much of their clinical business outside of primary care (e.g., Rich et al., 1995) or add new personnel to the primary care team (Litzelman et al., 1993).

The arguments for specialized geriatric care providers and teams are compelling, but their involvement in day-to-day geriatric care remains problematic. As discussed more thoroughly in the next chapter, the effectiveness of outpatient geriatric consultation remains unsettled. Should chronically ill seniors with multiple conditions receive care simultaneously from the diabetes clinical nurse, the congestive heart failure nurse specialist, and the disability prevention nurse? Some evidence suggests that most patients value their single source of usual care and that continuous primary care is cost-effective (Becker, Drachman, & Kirscht, 1974; Hjortdahl & Laerum, 1992; Wasson et al., 1984). Given the huge number of seniors and the chronically anemic supply of geriatricians, generalists will continue to provide the vast majority of medical care for seniors for the foreseeable future. How to utilize, maximally, our short supply of geriatricians to support primary care is an important unanswered question.

Can primary care be reoriented and reorganized to better meet the needs of the chronically ill older patient? Recent work is providing some preliminary evidence that geriatric patient needs can better be met if the primary care practice team organizes itself to the task, changes practice systems, and better uses all members of the practice team. For example, the mini-clinic, developed in Britain, changes the orientation and design of office practice, but does so periodically (Farmer & Coulter, 1990; Thorn & Watkins, 1982). In this model, a group of patients with similar needs are invited to participate in longer visits with the primary care practice team at regular intervals. Each visit includes an assessment, individual visits with various members of the practice team (physician, nurse, pharmacist) and relevant specialists, a group meeting, and systematic follow-up. We are currently testing the effectiveness of mini-clinics with frail elders and patients with diabetes in a randomized trial at Group Health Cooperative, Seattle, Washington.

Following similar logic, physicians developed the Cooperative Health Care Clinic (CHCC) model at Kaiser-Permanente in Colorado (Beck et al., 1997). CHCC patients (seniors with at least one chronic illness and high health care utilization) meet in groups of 15 to 20 on a monthly basis with their primary care physician, nurse, and other health professionals. The 150-minute sessions include guided interactive education, blood pressure checks and other health maintenance activities, opportunities for one-on-one interactions with health care team members, and group planning and socialization. Randomized trial findings revealed that CHCC patients were more satisfied, more up-to-date in their preventive care, and used some health services less than comparison patients. The model is being tested further and disseminated throughout the Kaiser system.

As discussed above, the assurance of regular follow-up is an essential feature of successful geriatric programs and practices, and telephone follow-up appears to be a notably cost-effective way to do it (Wasson et al., 1992). We have found that, unfortunately, many practices, especially in HMOs, do not have the systems in place to make large numbers of phone calls or send out reminder mailings that will assure that interactions with patients occur at planned intervals.

Decision Support

Available evidence suggests that generalist physicians are less aware of effective therapies for chronic diseases and disabilities than are specialists (Wagner et al., 1996a) and may be less oriented to assessing function and intervening to preserve or improve it. Thus, a high priority for primary care systems is to make explicit the elements of good chronic illness care through clinical policies and guidelines and to increase the geriatrics expertise available to the primary care team in caring for chronically ill seniors. The successful chronic disease management programs reviewed in this chapter almost invariably operate from a protocol or plan, which provides an explicit statement of what needs to be done for patients and at what intervals. Practice guidelines are no panacea, but evidence suggests that guidelines may be an important foundation when used as part of more comprehensive practice improvement interventions (Grimshaw & Russell, 1993). Interventions that incorporate guidelines into the fabric of practice (e.g., by delegation to office staff or through reminders to patients or providers) enhance the likelihood of behavior change.

Conventional geriatric consultation with written recommendations has generally proven to be ineffective in altering physician behaviors. More personal communication by telephone (Reuben et al., 1996; Vinicor et al., 1987), through specially trained local experts or "gurus" (Stuart et al., 1991) or by specialists seeing patients collaboratively in the primary care setting (Katon et al., 1995; McCulloch, Price, Hindmarsh, & Wagner, in press), would seem to be approaches more likely to succeed. A central feature of our efforts to improve diabetes care at Group Health Cooperative is the diabetes expert team consisting of a diabetologist and diabetes nurse educator (McCulloch et al., in press). They see patients jointly with primary care teams in their practices; the goals of these joint visits are to model planned diabetes care, educate about guidelines, and give advice about specific difficult patients. Prospective data suggest that primary care practitioners who participated in diabetes joint visits in 1995 were more compliant with diabetes practice guidelines in 1996. Such a role may be the most cost-effective way to use scarce geriatric personnel.

Organization of Care

The structure and strategies of the larger health care organization influence provider behavior, patient behavior, and the organization's capacity to improve its systems and its care. In addition to providing support to its constituent practices, the larger organization may be able to influence chronic illness care (for better or worse) by virtue of the incentives and regulations it imposes on its providers, the links it develops with key community resources, and the approaches it takes to quality improvement. Although strong empiric support is lacking, organizations that value and reward preventively oriented chronic illness care are likely to have better outcomes. Such rewards might include financial bonuses, reduced panel sizes, and additional staff as a result of better process and outcome measures. Links with high-quality community resources for important services such as support groups, transportation, and exercise programming would likely increase the appropriate use of such services.

Finally, some of the best intentioned efforts to improve chronic illness care have failed because most systems and practices don't have a built-in "capacity to change" (Carlson & Rosenqvist, 1991). For example, most practice teams don't have meetings that would allow them to consider the implementation of a new guideline, a new computer system, or the amelioration of a deficiency in care processes or outcomes. Team meetings have been found to be predictors of better care (Stason et al., 1994). Recent evidence suggests that the incorporation of modern quality improvement strategies into the day-to-day work of busy practices is possible and may be leading to valuable practice changes (Solberg, Mosser, & McDonald, 1997; Wasson, Jette, Johnson, Mohr, & Nelson, 1997). If health systems are going to improve outcomes in older persons with chronic illnesses, they must give their primary care practices the tools and the time to change the way they deliver care.

SUMMARY

Improving the care of a population of older persons with chronic illness will call for health care organizations to provide more than an assessment questionnaire or a few case managers. It requires a coherent strategy including a decision about the basic care model—bypass versus primary care (or an explicit compromise)—and a commitment to change incentives, develop links, and foster local quality improvement as well as to ensure the availability of guidelines, registries, self-management programs, and other critical elements. This will be aided by the selection or development of approaches that apply to multiple chronic illnesses. The technology to reduce mortality, dysfunction, and discomfort in most common chronic illnesses now exists. Getting this technology to all the relevant patients in a practice or health plan is the current challenge, and we now have proven approaches and models to begin to address this next set of challenges. It is time to get started.

REFERENCES

Anderson, R. M., Funnell, M. M., Butler, P. M., Arnold, M. S., Fitzgerald, J. T., & Feste, C. C. (1995). Patient empowerment: Results of a randomized controlled trial. *Diabetes Care, 18,* 943–949.

Beck, A., Scott, J., Williams, P., Robertson, B., Jackson, D., Gade, G., & Cowan, P. (1997). A randomized trial of group outpatient visits for chronically ill older HMO members: The cooperative health care clinic. *Journal of the American Geriatrics Society, 45,* 543–549.

Becker, M. H.. Drachman, R. H., & Kirscht, J. P. (1974). Continuity of pediatrician: New support for an old shobboleth. *Journal of Pediatrics, 84,* 599–605.

Bortz, W. M. II (1982). Disuse and aging. *Journal of the American Medical Association, 248,* 1203–1208.

Bruce, M. L., Seeman, T. E., Merrill, S. S., & Blazer, D. G. (1994). The impact of depressive symptomatology on physical disability: MacArthur studies of successful aging. *American Journal of Public Health, 84,* 1796–1799.

Buchner, D. M., & Wagner, E. H. (1992). Preventing frail health. *Clinics in Geriatric Medicine, 8,* 1–17.

Carlson, A., & Rosenqvist, U. (1991). Diabetes care organization, process, and patient outcomes: Effects of a diabetes control program. *Diabetes Education, 17*, 42–48.

Center for the Advancement of Health. (1996). An indexed bibliography on self-management for people with chronic disease. Washington, DC: Author.

Clark, N. M., Becker, M. H., Janz, N. K., Lorig, K., Rakowski, W., & Anderson, L. (1991). Self-management of chronic disease by older adults: A review and questions for research. *Journal of Aging and Health, 3*, 3–27.

Eisenberg, J. M. (1995). Commentary: Are differences in outcome due to differences in doctors or their patients? *Health Services Research, 30*, 291–294.

Ettinger, W. H., Jr., Fried, L. P., Harris, T., Shemanski, L., Shultz, R. J., for the CHS Collaborative Research Group. (1994). Self-reported causes of physical disability in older people: The Cardiovascular Health Study. *Journal of the American Geriatrics Society, 42*, 1035–1044.

Farmer, A., & Coulter, A. (1990). Organization of care for diabetic patients in general practice: Influence on hospital admissions. *British Journal of General Practitioners, 40*, 56–58.

Fry, J. (1973). Record keeping in primary care. In D. L. Sackett & M. S. Basking (Eds.), *Methods of health care evaluation* (2nd ed.). Hamilton, Ontario, Canada: McMaster University.

Greenfield, S., Kaplan, S. H., Ware, J. E., Yano, E. M., & Frank, H. J. L. (1988). Patients' participation in medical care: Effects on blood sugar control and quality of life in diabetes. *Journal of General Internal Medicine, 3*, 448–457.

Greenlick, M. R. (1992). Educating physicians for population-based clinical practice. *Journal of the American Medical Association, 267*, 1645–1648.

Grimshaw, J. M., & Russell, I. T. (1993). Effect of clinical guidelines on medical practice: A systematic review of rigorous evaluations. *Lancet, 342*, 1317–1322.

Guralnick, J. M., LaCroix, A. Z., Abbott, R. D., Berkman, L. F., Satterfield, S., Evans, D. A., & Wallace, R. B. (1993). Maintaining mobility in late life: Part 1. Demographic characteristics and chronic conditions. *American Journal of Epidemiology, 137*, 845–857.

Hampson, S. E., Glasgow, R. E., & Toobert, D. J. (1990). Personal models of diabetes and their relations to self-care activities. *Health Psychology, 9*, 632–646.

Hirsch, C. H., & Winograd, C. H., (1996). Clinic-based primary care of frail older patients in California. *Western Journal of Medicine, 156*, 385–391.

Hjortdahl, P., & Laerum, E. (1992). Continuity of care in general practice: Effect on patient satisfaction. *British Medical Journal, 304*, 1287–1290.

Johnston, M. E., Langton, K. B., Haynes, R. B., & Mathieu, A. (1994). Effects of computer-based clinical decision support systems on clinician performance and patient outcome: A critical appraisal of research. *Annals of Internal Medicine, 120*, 135–142.

Katon, W., Von Korff, M., Lin, E., Walker, E., Simon, G. E., Bush, T., Robinson, P., & Russo, J. (1995). Collaborative management to achieve treatment guidelines. *Journal of the American Medical Association, 273*, 1026–1031.

Kosorok, M. R., Omenn, G. S., Diehr, P., Koepsell, T. D., & Patrick, D. L. (1992). Restricted activity days among older adults. *American Journal of Public Health, 82*, 1263–1267.

Kottke, T. E., Brekke, M. L., & Solberg, L. L. (1993). Making "time" for preventive services. *Mayo Clinic Proceedings, 68,* 785–791.

Kriska, A. M., Baules, C., Cauley, J. A, LaPorte, R. E., Sandler, R. B., & Pambianco G. (1986). A randomized exercise trial in older women: Increased activity over two years and the factors associated with compliance. *Medicine and Science in Sports and Exercise, 18,* 557–562.

Krumholtz, H. M., Radford, M. J., Ellerback, E. F., Hennen, J., Meehan, T. P., Petrillo, M., Wang, Y., & Jencks, S. F. (1996). Aspirin for secondary prevention after acute myocardial infarction in the elderly: Prescribed use and outcomes. *Annals of Internal Medicine, 124,* 292–298.

Leveille, S. G., Wagner, E. H., Davis, C., Grothaus, L., Wallace, J., LoGerfo, M., & Kent, D. (1998). Preventing disability and managing chronic illness in frail older adults: A randomized trial of a community-based partnership with primary care. *Journal of the American Geriatrics Society, 46,* 1–9.

Litzelman, D. K., Slemenda, C. W., Langefield, C. D., Hays, L. M., Welch, M. A., Bild, D. E., Ford, E. S., & Vinicor, F. (1993). Reduction of lower extremity clinical abnormalities in patients with non-insulin-dependent diabetes mellitus: A randomized controlled trial. *Annals of Internal Medicine, 119,* 36–41.

Lorig, K., & Holman, H. (1993). Arthritis self-management studies: A 12-year review. *Health-Education Quarterly, 20,* 17–28.

Lorig, K., Holman, H. R., Sobel, D., Laurenti, D., Gonzalez, V., & Minor, M. (1994). Living a healthy life with chronic conditions. Palo Alto, CA: Bull Publishing.

Maisiak, R., Austin, J., & Heck, L. (1996). Health outcomes of two telephone interventions for patients with rheumatoid arthritis or osteoarthritis. *Arthritis and Rheumatism, 39,* 1391–1399.

Maki, B. E., Holliday, P. J., & Topper, A. K. (1991). Fear of falling and postural performance in the elderly. *Journal of Gerontology, 46,* M123–M131.

McCulloch, D. K., Price, M. J., Hindmarsh, M., & Wagner, E. H. (in press). Implementation of a comprehensive program to promote a population-based approach to diabetes management in a primary care setting: Early results and lessons learned. *Effective Clinical Practice.*

Montgomery, E. B. J., Lieberman, A., Singh, G., & Fries, J. F. (1994). Patient education and health promotion can be effective in Parkinson's disease: A randomized controlled trial. PROPATH Advisory Board [see comments]. *American Journal of Medicine, 97,* 429–435.

Moore, A. A., & Siu, A. L. (1996). Screening for common problems in ambulatory elderly: Clinical confirmation of a screening instrument. American Journal of Medicine, 100, 438–443.

Reuben, D. B., Maly, R. C., Hirsch, S. H., Frank, J. C., Oakes, A. M., Siu, A. L., & Hays, R. D. (1996). Physician implementation of and patient adherence to recommendations from comprehensive geriatric assessment. *American Journal of Medicine, 100,* 444–451.

Rich, M. W., Beckham, V., Wittenberg, C., Leven, C. L., Freedland, K. E., & Carney, R. M. (1995). A multidisciplinary intervention to prevent the readmission of elderly patients with congestive heart failure. *New England Journal of Medicine, 333,* 1190–1195.

Rich, M. W., Vinson, J. M., Sperry J. C., Shah, A. S., Spinner, L. R., Chung, M. K., &

Davila-Roman, V. (1993). Prevention of readmission in elderly patients with congestive heart failure: Results of a prospective, randomized pilot study. *Journal of General Internal Medicine, 8*, 585–590.

Solberg, L. I., Mosser, G., & McDonald, S. (1997). The three faces of performance measurement: Improvement, accountability, and research. *Joint Commission Journal on Quality Improvement, 23*, 135–147.

Stason W. B., Shepard, D. S., Perry, Jr, H. M., Carmen, B. M., Nagurney, J. T., Rosner, B., & Meyer, G. (1994). Effectiveness and costs of veterans affairs hypertension clinic. *Medical Care, 32*, 1197–1215.

Stuart, M. E., Handley M. A, Chamberlain M. A., Wallach, R. W., Penna, P. M., & Stergachis, A. (1991). Successful implementation of a guideline program for the rational use of lipid-lowering drugs. *HMO Practice, 5*, 198–204.

Thorn, P. A., & Watkins, P. (1982). Organization of diabetic care. *British Medical Journal, 285*, 787–789.

Vinicor, F., Cohen, S. J., Mazzuca, S. A., Moorman, N., Wheeler, M., Kuebler, T., Swanson, S., Ours, P., Fineberg, S. E., Gordon, E. E., Duckworth, W., Norton, J. A., Fineberg, N. S., & Clark, C. M., Jr. (1987). DIABEDS: A randomized trial of the effects of physician and/or patient education on diabetes patient outcomes. *Journal of Chronic Diseases, 40*, 345–356.

Von Korff, M., Gruman, J., Schaefer, J., Curry, S., & Wagner, E. H. (1997). Collaborative management of chronic illness: Essential elements. *Annals of Internal Medicine, 127* 1097–1102.

Wagner, E. H. (1995). Population-based management of diabetes care. *Patient Education Counseling, 26*, 225–230.

Wagner, E. H. (1997). Managed care and chronic illness: Health services research needs. *Health Services Research, 32*, 702–714.

Wagner, E. H. (1996). The promise and performance of HMOs in improving outcomes in older adults. *Journal of the American Geriatrics Society, 44*, 1–7.

Wagner, E. H., Austin, A., & Von Korff, M. (1996a). Organizing care for patients with chronic illness. *Milbank Quarterly, 74*, 1–34.

Wagner, E. H., Austin, B., & Von Korff, M. (1996b). Improving outcomes in chronic illness. *Managed Care Quarterly, 4*, 12–25.

Wagner, E. H., LaCroix A. Z., Buchner, D. M., & Larson, E. B. (1992). Effects of physical activity on health status in older adults: Part 1. Observational studies. *Annual Review of Public Health, 13*, 451–468.

Wagner, E. H., LaCroix, A. Z., Grothaus, L., Leveille, S. G., Hecht, J. A., Artz, K., Odle, K., & Buchner, D. M. (1994). Preventing disability and falls in older adults: A population-based randomized trial. *American Journal of Public Health, 84*, 1800–1806.

Wallace, J. I., Buchner, D. M., Grothaus, L., Leveille, S., LaCroix, A. Z., & Wagner, E. H. (1998). Implementation and effectiveness of a community-based health promotion program for older adults. *Journals of Gerontology, 53A*, M301–M306.

Wasson, J., Gaudette, C., Whaley, F., Sauvigne, A., Baribeau, P., & Welch, H. G. (1992). Telephone care as a substitute for routine clinic follow-up [see comments]. *Journal of the American Medical Association, 267*, 1788–1793.

Wasson, J. H., Sauvigne, A. E., Mogielnicki, R. P., Frey, W. G., Sox, C. H., Gandette,

C., & Trockwell, A. (1984). Continuity of outpatient medical care in elder men: A randomized trial. *Journal of the American Medical Association, 252,* 2413–2417.

Wasson, J. H., Jette, A. M., Johnson, D. J., Mohr, J. J., & Nelson, E. C. (1997). A replicable and customizable approach to improve ambulatory care and research. *Journal of Ambulatory Care Management, 20,* 17–27.

Wells, K. B., Katon, W., Rogers, B., & Camp P. (1994). Use of minor tranquilizers and antidepressant medications by depressed outpatients: Results from the Medical Outcomes Study. *American Journal of Psychiatry, 151,* 694–700.

4

Care of Older People at Risk

Chad Boult and James T. Pacala

Most seniors are healthy, but a minority have chronic conditions that require frequent, intensive, and expensive care. As a result, 5% to 10% of seniors consistently incur 60% to 70% of the older population's annual health care expenses (Freeborn, Pope, Mullooly, & McFarland, 1990; Gornick, McMillan, & Lubitz, 1993; Gruenberg, Tompkins, & Porell, 1989). This dense concentration of morbidity and use of health-related services is unfortunate for those afflicted, but it offers hope for effectively focusing resources where they will do the most good. This chapter begins by describing currently available methods for identifying high-risk seniors (i.e., those whose chronic conditions place them at risk for developing health-related crises and for needing expensive health care). It then discusses several options for reducing risk, presenting the available data about the outcomes and cost-effectiveness of these approaches. The conclusion makes recommendations for implementing these interventions within today's (and tomorrow's) systems of health care for older persons.

In a capitated environment, organizations bearing financial risk for the health care of older populations have strong financial incentives to identify high-risk persons as promptly as possible and then to provide them special care designed to optimize their health and avert future health-related crises. Such a long-term investment strategy is feasible because most seniors do not change health care systems often; disenrollment from Medicare HMOs averages less than 8% per year (Nelson et al., 1996). If successful, this strategy would lead to better quality of life, higher levels of satisfaction with care, and lower total costs for many high-risk older persons. We should recognize, however, that early detection may not be cost-effective for all high-risk conditions and that not every senior wants intervention.

Nevertheless, these incentives, coupled with the availability of pooled capitation dollars, are nudging health care organizations to invest increasingly in innovative systems of care for high-risk seniors. Organizations can deliver some new programs to large numbers of seniors at relatively low per capita cost (e.g., self-management programs, group activities, and messages in popular media). The more intensive programs probably need to focus selectively—if they are to be cost-effective—on those most likely to benefit. The available evidence about the cost-effectiveness of interventions for at-risk seniors warrants a hard look.

IDENTIFYING HIGH-RISK SENIORS

The initial challenge is to anticipate which high-risk persons would be appropriate recipients of the more intensive interventions (i.e., seniors whose health-related problems are likely to lead to expensive crises but could be ameliorated by special care). Organizations currently use three complementary approaches to identify these persons: periodic screening of the population by mail or telephone, recognition by clinicians, and analysis of administrative data (see Figure 4.1). None of these approaches is sufficient as a single method. Surveys are superficial, incomplete (<100% response rates), and only moderately accurate; clinicians may lack expertise, incentive, or regular contact with many seniors; administrative data reflect primarily the past and are often not readily accessible. The ideal monitoring system would integrate data from all three sources.

Clinicians and researchers have created and applied many screening tools for estimating the risk of undesirable outcomes in ambulatory populations (Brody, Johnson, & Ried, 1997; Coleman, Grothaus, Buchner, Hecht, & Wagner, 1997; Freedman, Beck, Robertson, Calonge, & Gade, 1996) and in hospitalized patients (Reuben et al., 1992; Sager et al., 1996). Other tools identify seniors at risk for specific conditions (e.g., osteoporosis, falls, poor nutrition, and depression). The most extensively studied and widely used general screening instrument consists of eight questions that surveyors ask by mail or by telephone (see list in Appendix A) (Boult et al., 1993). Analysis of the responses using a formula, shown in Appendix B, produces an estimate of the probability of repeated admission (P_{ra}) to a hospital in the future. P_{ra} values above a predetermined threshold indicate a high-risk status and a need for further evaluation.

Longitudinal studies have shown that seniors' risk status often changes over time; 15% to 20% of functionally disabled older persons regain their independence within a year. Nevertheless, prospective testing of the P_{ra} instrument in three diverse populations has confirmed that high-risk seniors use twice as many health-related services as low-risk seniors during the 1 to 4 years after they complete the eight questions (see Table 4.1) (Boult et al., 1993; Pacala, Boult, & Boult, 1995; Pacala, Boult, Reed, & Aliberti, 1997).

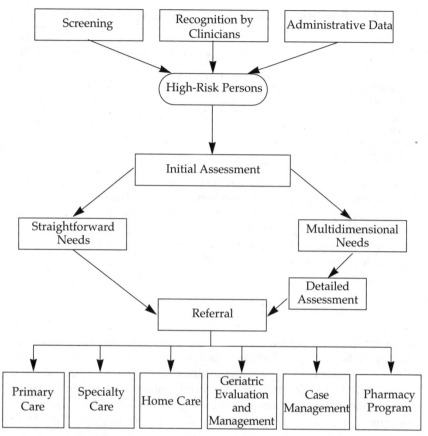

FIGURE 4.1 **Identification and management of high-risk seniors.**

The implementation of a risk-monitoring program, even if limited to the use of an eight-item questionnaire, is a multifaceted challenge that requires careful planning and budgeting. At a minimum, it requires an ongoing system of data collection, entry, management, analysis, and reporting. Organizations willing to make significant investments in hardware, software, and personnel may wish to conduct their own screening programs. Others may wish to contract with data management companies that will conduct parts or all of the screening process.

The design, initiation, and maintenance of more comprehensive risk-monitoring systems demand even more resources. These systems may include "hot lines" for clinicians to identify high-risk patients and computer programs that electronically scan administrative databases (Coleman et al., 1997) to identify seniors who have ominous diagnoses, medication profiles, or patterns of using health-related services (e.g., emergency rooms).

TABLE 4.1 Predictive Accuracy of P$_{ra}$ Screening Instrument

	Low Risk	High Risk	Ratio (High/Low)	Date Data Acquired
Annual Hospital Days				
National Medicare population	2.6	5.2	2.0	1984–1988
Local Medicaid population	2.4	4.5	1.9	1992–1993
Annual HMO Costs				
California HMO	$1,331	$2,756	2.1	1991-1993
· (costs of noncapitated care)				

On a cautionary note, we should acknowledge that the cost-effectiveness of "targeting" (focusing intensive interventions on the high-risk minority of the older population) is still debated. The weight of the evidence supports the value of targeting, but no studies have directly compared the outcomes of intensive interventions for targeted populations versus non-targeted populations.

ASSESSING HIGH-RISK SENIORS

Following their identification, high-risk seniors often receive some sort of special care to alter their health careers favorably. The first logical step, a brief initial assessment, aims to determine the complexity of the identified person's needs and to arrange appropriate follow-up care. In some programs, an experienced nurse conducts a brief, semi-structured initial assessment interview, either in person or by telephone. The HMO Workgroup on Care Management recently published a suggested set of interview questions and a guide to the interpretation of seniors' responses (Aliotta et al., 1997).

The initial assessment interview will determine that some seniors are not at high risk after all; that is, they are false positives from the risk-identification process or have problems that cannot be modified. Interviewers will find that other seniors have straightforward needs that can be met by providing information or by making a referral. The remaining seniors, those with high but potentially modifiable risks, have complex needs requiring more in-depth evaluation leading to comprehensive plans of action.

A team—either interdisciplinary or multidisciplinary—usually performs a comprehensive assessment of this last group, although innovative approaches are challenging this axiom (Leveille et al., 1997). Teams typically consist of a physician, a nurse, and/or a social worker, all of whom have expertise in the care of older adults. Each member meets individually with the patient to evaluate the issues specific to his or her discipline that have surfaced during the risk-identification and initial assessment processes. This comprehensive geriatric assessment (CGA) is a diagnostic process intended to determine the person's medical, psychosocial, and functional capabilities and limitations in order to develop an overall plan for treatment and long-term follow-up (Rubenstein, Stuck, Siu, & Wieland, 1991). Appendix C provides examples of the instruments frequently used to evaluate the major health-related domains. In interdisciplinary teams, the team members meet after their individual data-gathering encounters to establish priorities, to plan care, and to take responsibility for specific next steps. In multidisciplinary teams, each professional prepares a separate set of recommendations.

CGA focuses on assessing elders' problems and recommending treatments, but it leaves interventions to other health care providers. Several studies have shown that CGA, although helpful in diagnosis, has not consistently improved patient outcomes (Solomon, 1988), perhaps because only 50% to 70% of its recommendations have been implemented (Cefalu, Kaslow, Mims, & Simpson, 1995; Epstein et al., 1990; Shah, Maly, Frank, Hirsch, & Reuben, 1997). However, more recent efforts to improve the follow-up communication about CGA recommendations with primary physicians, patients, and families have increased the proportion of implemented recommendations to about 80% (Reuben et al.,1997).

The assessment process often reveals a myriad of health-related problems. Unfortunately, many present assessment programs do not delineate in advance the priorities and the processes used in planning care, so the plans and their effectiveness vary from program to program. Recent work has begun to identify the conditions on which teams might best focus their efforts (i.e., the conditions that often lead to the greatest losses and costs and for which treatment is the most effective). For example, research has found that impairments in vision, hearing, lower extremity strength, and affect are precursors of falls, incontinence, and functional dependency (Tinetti, Inouye, Gill, & Doucette, 1995). Validated instruments are available to detect these and other sentinel conditions (e.g., poor nutrition, cognitive impairment) (Moore & Siu, 1996), and evidence-based guidelines for effective treatment are becoming available. The assessment programs of the future would do well to set clinical priorities and plan care on the basis of emerging evidence indicating which interventions are the most beneficial.

MANAGING HIGH-RISK SENIORS

As systems of health care become more sophisticated, the number and range of interventions available to high-risk seniors through CGA and other channels will grow. The following pages describe some of the more promising interventions and summarize the existing evidence of their effectiveness.

Geriatric Evaluation and Management

Early studies showed that CGA is most likely to improve patients' functional status if the clinicians who implement its recommendations have control of their care (Applegate & Burns, 1996; Burns, 1994). The expanded process is geriatric evaluation and management (GEM). A recent meta-analysis of 28 CGA and GEM programs confirmed that most effective programs combine assessment with sustained control over management (Rubenstein, Bernabei, & Wieland, 1994; Stuck, Siu, Wieland, & Rubenstein, 1993).

Although some of the most successful outcomes from GEM have occurred in inpatient settings (Rubenstein et al., 1984), the cost of such interventions is high, encouraging the delivery of GEM in less expensive outpatient settings. Unfortunately, the overall results of most published studies of outpatient GEM have been inconsistent and disappointing. Individual controlled trials, however, have demonstrated GEM's potential to improve a variety of outcomes within the outpatient setting; Table 4.2 lists examples. Characteristics common to the outpatient GEM programs that have produced positive results include

- the targeting of patients who are neither too healthy nor too sick to benefit
- the use of carefully selected standard assessment instruments
- small close-knit teams of clinicians who are trained and interested in geriatrics
- effective communication with patients, families, and primary care physicians
- treatment for several months according to well-established principles of geriatrics

Case Management

Only a small percentage (perhaps 20%) of seniors initially identified as high risk have combinations of treatable conditions so complex that the benefits of sustained team management outweigh the costs. The other 80% have needs that are either straightforward, unresponsive to presently available treatments, or best managed by their own primary care physicians—or they do not wish to accept care from a GEM team. Many high-risk seniors who are not appropriate recipients of GEM (and most who are) may benefit from case management (CM). Case managers, whose

TABLE 4.2   Individual Controlled Trials Showing Improved Outcomes From Outpatient GEM

Positive Outcome Associated With Outpatient GEM	Authors	Years
Improved diagnostic accuracy	Silverman et al.	1995
	Tulloch & Moore	1979
Improved functional ability	Williams et al.	1987
	Yeo et al.	1987
Increased satisfaction with care	Engelhardt et al.	1996
Increased use of home services	Williams et al.	1987
	Yeo et al.	1987
	Rubin et al.	1992
	Rubin et al.	1993
Decreased mortality	Toseland et al.	1996
Decreased health care costs	Tulloch & Moore	1979
	Williams et al.	1987
	Rubin et al.	1992
Decreased patient anxiety	Silverman et al.	1995
	Toseland et al.	1996
Decreased depression	Toseland et al.	1996
	Burns et al.	1995
Decreased stress for caregivers	Silverman et al.	1995
Decreased use of emergency services	Engelhardt et al.	1996
Decreased use of hospital services	Tulloch & Moore	1979
	Williams et al.	1987
	Rubin et al.	1992

backgrounds are usually in nursing or social work, arrange social and health-related services and coordinate these services across a wide range of settings (Kodner, 1993).

A 1994 survey found that all large Medicare HMOs offer some form of CM that involves many, and often all, of the following processes: case finding, assessing clients' needs, planning their care, implementing plans, and monitoring the care provided (Pacala et al., 1995). Most HMOs reported that they designed their CM programs to reduce hospital use, increase enrollee and provider satisfaction, and optimize the functional ability of their enrollees. Although many HMO executives reported decreased hospitalization among enrollees who received CM, few provided data to support these claims. Nevertheless, most asserted they were committed to continuing or expanding their CM programs.

Most CM programs are one of two types. In low-volume and high-intensity programs, the case managers carry caseloads of 60 or fewer clients, see these clients frequently, and both provide and arrange services for them. In high-volume and low-intensity programs, the case managers arrange services for 100 or more clients but see them infrequently. Unfortunately, CM programs are extremely heterogeneous, and many are loosely structured. The case managers receive variable amounts of training, the criteria for offering CM to clients may be subjective, and the services provided may not consistently focus on activities that are likely to yield maximal benefit. Some programs emphasize cost containment more than risk reduction.

When interviewed anonymously, case managers and their supervisors state that effective case management results from clear role definitions; a team approach with good communication; formulation of specific, realistic individual plans of care; strong organizational support; and enrollees', physicians', and family members' familiarity with and acceptance of CM (Pacala & Boult, 1996).

The first randomized trial of CM targeted seniors who were hospitalized with congestive heart failure (CHF). Before discharge, the patients received intensive, structured education about CHF from a nurse and a dietitian. Their discharge arrangements and postdischarge services, arranged and coordinated by a social worker, included home care and telephone follow-up. During the 90 days after discharge, recipients of CM, compared with recipients of usual care, had 56.2% fewer hospital admissions, slightly lower costs of care, and twice as much improvement in quality of life scores (Rich et al., 1995). In contrast, a less structured, less proactive form of CM, when appraised by a randomized trial, led to increased use of hospitals and no improvement in quality of life (Weinberger, Oddonne, & Henderson, 1996). Additional randomized trials of various forms of CM are now under way.

In programs of the future, adherence to the principles illustrated by the CHF-CM study above would probably maximize the benefits of CM: systematic targeting, clear roles and treatment protocols, proactive follow-up, and patient self-management.

Interdisciplinary Home Care

A related intervention for some functionally disabled seniors is to provide physician-led interdisciplinary home care (IHC). The integration of medical and supportive services distinguishes IHC from other forms of home care in which communication between physicians and other home care providers is usually limited to the exchange of written notes and authorizations. IHC attempts to minimize morbidity and mortality and maximize the older person's ability to live in the community as long as possible.

Case managers may initiate, coordinate, or even partially provide these services. In IHC, nurses monitor seniors' ability to live independently, suggest changes in supportive and therapeutic services, evaluate home safety, educate patients and their families, and reinforce the principles of self-care. Home health aides provide personal care and homemaker services. Occupational and physical therapists provide rehabilitative services as needed. Occasional home visits by physicians, though not at first glance cost-effective, can obviate the need for the expensive, labor-intensive, uncomfortable, and sometimes disorienting transportation of frail elders to physicians' offices. IHC teams meet regularly to discuss their cases.

As shown in Table 4.3 all three published randomized clinical trials of IHC suggest that, unlike traditional forms of home care (Hedrick & Inui, 1986; Weissert & Hedrick, 1994), IHC may be cost-effective (Cummings et al., 1990; Melin, Hakansson, & Bygren, 1993; Zimmer, Groth-Juncker, & McCusker, 1985). In each of the IHC programs studied, the intervention was provided only to functionally disabled seniors and was characterized by leadership of the team by a home care physician, education and support of the family caregivers, and regular team conferences. After 6 months, receiving IHC was associated with significantly greater use of in-home services and greater satisfaction with care by the family caregivers—and with consistent trends toward lower use of clinics, institutional services, and total resources. In the two programs in which the patients were highly disabled or terminal and in which the IHC physicians managed all hospital as well as home care, the trends toward cost savings resulted from fewer hospital days. In the other program, which excluded severely disabled patients, significant cost savings resulted from greater functional improvement and fewer nursing home days. The effectiveness of IHC under other conditions (e.g., capitated reimbursement, patients with minor disabilities, and teams led by patients' regular primary physicians) has yet to be tested.

In spite of these data, the medical and supportive components of home care in the United States are rarely well integrated. Home health services for Medicare beneficiaries are used for long-term supportive care much more than for medical management, and there is a large geographic variation in the use of these services (Welch, Wennberg, & Welch, 1996). The rapidly increasing use of these nonintegrated, supportive home health services, coupled with a lack of data about their effectiveness, has prompted federal officials to reconsider the criteria under which Medicare will cover traditional home health services. Chapters 5 and 12 more fully describe home care as a method for treating acute illness and long-term disability.

Disease Management Programs

Disease management programs that provide comprehensive care for specific illnesses have proliferated recently. Often provider organizations

TABLE 4.3 Studies of Interdisciplinary Home Care

Author	Year	Country	Intervention	Design	Significant* Results Associated With Interdisciplinary Home Care	Control
Mitchell	1978	U.S.	Home care by interdisciplinary team	Quasi-experimental ($n = 318$)	Better functional ability; lower rate of hospital admissions (12% vs. 28%)	Nursing home care
Zimmer et al.	1985	U.S.	Home care by interdisciplinary team	RCT** ($n = 167$)	More home services; higher satisfaction by informal caregivers	Physician care
Cummings et al.	1990	U.S.	Home care by interdisciplinary team	RCT ($n = 419$)	Higher satisfaction by informal caregivers; lower 6-month mean hospital costs ($3,000 vs. $4,246)	Usual care in Veterans Administration
Challis et al.	1991	U.K.	Home care by interdisciplinary team	Quasi-experimental ($n = 214$)	Better morale and affect	Nursing home care or day hospital
Melin et al.	1993	Sweden	Home care by interdisciplinary team	RCT ($n = 183$)	Better functional ability; fewer drugs; fewer unresolved diagnoses; 67% fewer mean nursing home days	Home care by usual caregivers

* $p < 0.05$
** Randomized controlled trial

74

offer these services to HMOs for the benefit of their members. These "carve-out" interventions for treating such chronic conditions as emphysema, diabetes, mental illness, and cancer may benefit some high-risk older people who have only one serious problem and are otherwise healthy. Unfortunately, the typical high-risk senior has a complex combination of chronic conditions that, under a disease management model of care, might require several disease management programs, several teams of providers, and probably several case managers. Integration of such care would be seriously problematic. Data about the effects of disease management programs on high-risk older populations have yet to be published in the peer-reviewed scientific literature.

RECOMMENDATIONS

Many organized systems of health care now monitor the risk status of their senior populations and provide high-risk members with some form of case management. Far fewer offer interdisciplinary home care, GEM, or other proactive interventions, partly because evidence of cost-effectiveness is lacking, and partly because geriatricians and gerontological nurse practitioners (NPs) are scarce. In the future, data, vision, and market forces will influence the evolution of new systems of care.

Specific Programs

As of 1998, the data describing the effectiveness and the costs of most of the programs described in this chapter are incomplete; they do not allow leaders to make decisions easily about implementing new initiatives. A few efforts to measure the cost-effectiveness of these innovative programs are under way, but hundreds of experimental programs are being fielded without well-designed evaluative components. When data about programs' effects on health status, functional ability, satisfaction with care, and use of health-related services eventually become available, decisions about system development can rest more heavily on evidence.

The data now available about the outcomes of interventions for high-risk older persons most strongly support the implementation of interdisciplinary home care and structured case management for congestive heart failure. Additional data about the cost-effectiveness of GEM and CM will emerge in the next few years.

In using these data to select innovations for future implementation, organizations would be wise to ensure that the tested interventions under consideration are standardized and explicit. Attempting to replicate a concept is a risky new experiment unto itself. Similarly, all of the interventions described above have various configurations. The saying "If you've seen one CM program, you've seen one CM program" attests to the wide heterogeneity among the tactics of CM programs operating today. Before investing in the implementation of any previously tested program for high-risk seniors, organizations should carefully investigate the feasibility of reproducing the exact methods locally that led to good outcomes elsewhere.

As we look across the successful innovations in the care of high-risk seniors, a few common elements emerge: targeting services to those most likely to benefit; developing well-trained interdisciplinary teams of professional caregivers; performing focused, standardized assessments; providing proactive, goal-oriented, protocol-driven care; telephoning patients to follow up on recommended regimens; and promoting seniors' and families' involvement in their own care. In the years ahead, new types of programs for delivering these (and other) elements will probably evolve and be even more effective than today's best programs. Ultimately, mature systems of health care will likely incorporate such "elements of success" into a wide range of services for high-risk older persons. Comprehensive delivery systems that offer most (if not all) of the successful elements and programs described above will meet the needs of this population most effectively and efficiently.

Organized systems that invest in special programs for high-risk seniors must learn to integrate those programs so as not to overwhelm these seniors or lose them to systemic oblivion. Organizations should avoid and prevent fragmentation of care, the Achilles' heel of our present system of care for persons with complex needs. The cornerstone of integration will probably be good primary care, in which one provider, collaborating with other professionals and special services, oversees all of an older person's care.

Decisions about implementing programs for high-risk seniors will also reflect executives' vision of their organizations' mission. Those who equate future success with an ability to enhance health, and thereby to contain costs, are likely to invest in proactive preventive programs. Those who seek more immediate financial returns are likely to invest more heavily in marketing, utilization management, and programs that reduce the costs of acute illness. Ultimately, market forces will probably determine the future. The prevention-oriented organizations will reap rewards for their investments to the extent that seniors and their families, through political and commercial channels, demand high-quality, health-sustaining care. Alternatively, the organizations seeking immediate returns will prosper to the extent that consumers' choices are influenced more by premiums and advertising.

Infrastructural Changes

The ability to implement many of the programs designed for high-risk seniors will depend on increased access to coordinated teams of clinical specialists (e.g., geriatricians, gerontological NPs, social workers, therapists, and other technicians), improved processes for educating primary providers about geriatrics, better alignment of incentives, and new integrated clinical information systems.

Many of the interventions described earlier rely on teams of professionals with expertise in geriatrics. The creation of effective interdisciplinary teams requires time, training, communication, and the revision of many traditional roles. Professionals from different disciplines must learn each other's language, values, background, skills, and work habits. They must learn to respect, appreciate, and rely on each other. Attainment of such collaborative relationships will require commitment, resources, explicit training in team development, and patience—from our medical education system and from our health care organizations.

Establishing a cadre of skillful primary providers will also present a challenge. Many physicians, nurses, and other providers will need new knowledge, skills, and attitudes in order to practice effectively in the envisioned systems of the future. Case managers have identified physicians' lack of understanding of CM as one of the greatest barriers to its effectiveness (Pacala & Boult, 1996). Medical educators will need to upgrade traditional curricular components, such as courses, readings, and conferences, as they refine newer, more effective learning media such as on-line decision support and evidence-based practice guidelines. In the near future, quick access to consulting geriatricians by telephone or by two-way video communication (which allows consultants to interview and "examine" patients from afar) could improve primary care, while providing continuing education to practicing family physicians and general internists. However, the present shortage of geriatricians challenges the dissemination of even this high-efficiency model. The shortage of geriatric expertise, which is projected to increase in the coming years (Reuben et al., 1993), will command critical consideration in planning all future systems of health care for high-risk seniors. The curricula of most health professional schools and residency programs also need to emphasize more strongly the care of chronically ill older persons (Health Resources and Services Administration, 1995). Curricula and educational systems for training case managers are still in their infancy.

These programs of the future will require comprehensive, integrated information systems to facilitate many of the embedded processes: the screening of populations, the monitoring of individuals' risk levels, and the sharing of up-to-date clinical information among providers. Effective care coordination will require that basic clinical information be accessible on-line to providers at widely dispersed sites of care.

As systems of care become larger and more complex, it will also become increasingly important that they create and maintain incentives that encourage all of the participants to strive toward the global goals of the organization. Success will be more likely when they reward rather than penalize hospitals for cooperating with organizational initiatives to reduce hospital days, when they allow providers sufficient time and resources for planning and coordinating the care of their complex frail older patients, and when they reward providers to the extent that their efforts lead to desirable health outcomes and appropriate use of resources. Realigning incentives in large complex organizations is a long, tedious, often contentious process, yet one that will determine the ultimate success of implementing most of the interventions described in the preceding pages. Underlying the success of this realignment process is the need to link, if not merge, several diverse cultures: management, health care, science, and finance. The challenges will be at least as great as the potential rewards.

REFERENCES

Aliotta, S., Boult, C., Butin, D., Clark, J., Derouin, P., Fillet, H., Jenson, G., Pacala, J., Santa, J., Venohr, I., & Euchner, N. (1997). *Planning care for high-risk Medicare HMO members.* Washington, DC: AAHP Foundation.

Applegate, W., & Burns, R. (1996). Geriatric medicine. *Journal of the American Medical Association, 275,* 1812–1813.

Boult, C., Dowd, B., McCaffrey, D., Boult, L., Hernandez, R., & Krulewitch, H. (1993). Screening elders for risk of hospital admission. *Journal of the American Geriatrics Society, 41,* 811–817.

Brody, K. K., Johnson, R. E., & Ried, L. D. (1997). Evaluation of a self-report screening instrument to predict frailty outcomes in aging populations. *Gerontologist, 37,* 182–191.

Burns, R. (1994). Beyond the black box of comprehensive geriatric assessment. *Journal of the American Geriatrics Society, 42,* 1130.

Cefalu, C. A., Kaslow, L. D., Mims, B., & Simpson, S. (1995). Follow-up of comprehensive geriatric assessment in a family medicine residency clinic. *Journal of the American Board of Family Practice, 8,* 263–269.

Coleman, E. A., Grothaus, L. C., Buchner, D. M., Hecht, J. A., & Wagner, E. H. (1997). A comparison of models to predict hospitalization and functional decline (abstract). *Journal of the American Geriatrics Society, 45,* S55.

Cummings, J. E., Hughes, S. L., Weaver, F. M., Manheim, F. M., Conrad, K. J., Nash, K., Braun, B., & Adelman, J. (1990). Cost-effectiveness of Veterans Administration hospital-based home care: A randomized controlled trial. *Archives of Internal Medicine, 150,* 1274–1280.

Duke University. (1978). Multidimensional Functional Assessment: The OARS Methodology. Durham, NC: Duke University.

Epstein, A. M., Hall, J. A., Fretwell, M., Feldstein, M., DeCiantis, M. L., Tognetti, J., Cutler, C., Constantine, M., Besdine, R., Rowe, J., & McNeil, B. J. (1990). Consultative geriatric assessment of ambulatory patients. *Journal of the American Medical Association, 263,* 538–544.

Folstein, M. F., Folstein, S. E., & McHugh, P. R. (1975). Mini-mental state: A Practical method for grading the cognitive state of patients for the clinician. *Journal of Psychiatric Research, 12,* 189–198.

Freeborn, D. K., Pope, C. R., Mullooly, J. P., & McFarland, B. H. (1990). Consistently high users of medical care among the elderly. *Medical Care, 28,* 527–540.

Freedman, J. D., Beck, A., Robertson, B., Calonge, B. N., & Gade, G. (1996). Using a mailed survey to predict hospital admission among patients older than eighty. *Journal of the American Geriatrics Society, 44,* 689–692.

Gornick, M., McMillan, A., & Lubitz, J. (1993). A longitudinal perspective on patterns of Medicare payments. *Health Affairs, 12,* 140–150.

Gruenberg, L., Tompkins, C., & Porell, F. (1989). The health status and utilization patterns of the elderly: Implications for setting Medicare payments to HMOs. *Advances in Health Economics and Health Services Research, 10,* 41–73.

Health Resources and Services Administration. (1995). A national agenda for geriatric education: White papers. Washington, DC: U.S. Government Printing Office.

Hedrick, S. C., & Inui, T. S. (1986). The effectiveness and cost of home care: An information synthesis. *Health Services Review, 20,* 851–880.

Katz, S., Ford, A. B., Moskowitz, R. W., Jackson, B. A., & Jaffe, M. W. (1963). Studies of illness in the aged. The index of ADL: A standardized measure of biological and psychological function. *Journal of the American Medical Association, 185,* 914–919.

Kodner, D. L. (1993). *Case management: Principles, Practice and performance.* New York: Institute for Applied Gerontology.

Leveille, S. G., Wagner, E. H., Davis, C., Grothaus, L., Wallace, J., LoGerfo, M., & Kent, D. Preventing disability and managing chronic illness in frail older adults: A randomized trial of a community-based partnership with primary care. Manuscript submitted for publication.

Lubben, J. E. (1988). Assessing social networks among elderly populations. *Family and Community Health, 11,* 42–52.

Mayfield, D., McLeod, G., & Hall, P. (1974). The CAGE questionnaire: Validation of a new alcoholism screening instrument. *American Journal of Psychiatry, 131,* 1121–1123.

Melin, A., Hakansson, S., & Bygren, L. (1993). The cost and effectiveness of rehabilitation in the home: A study of Swedish elderly. *American Journal of Public Health, 83,* 356–362.

Moore, A. A., & Siu, A. L. (1996). Screening for common problems in ambulatory elderly: Clinical confirmation of a screening instrument. *American Journal of Medicine, 100,* 383–385.

Nelson, L., Gold, M., Brown, R., Ciemnecki, A. B., Aizer, A., & Cybulski, K. A. (1996). Access to care in Medicare managed care: Results from a 1996 survey of enrollees and disenrollees (Selected External Research Series No. 7). Washington, DC: Physician Payment Review Commission.

Pacala, J. T., & Boult, C. (1996). Factors influencing the effectiveness of case management in managed care organizations: A qualitative analysis. *Journal of Care Management, 2,* 29–35.

Pacala, J. T., Boult, C., & Boult, L. (1995). Predictive validity of a questionnaire that identifies elders at risk for hospital admission. *Journal of the American Geriatrics Society, 43,* 374–377.

Pacala, J. T., Boult, C., Hepburn, K., Kane, R. A., Kane, R. L., Malone, J., Morishita, L., & Reed, R. (1995). Case management of older adults in health maintenance organizations. *Journal of the American Geriatrics Society, 43,* 538–542.

Pacala, J. T., Boult, C., Reed, R. L., & Aliberti, E. (1997). Predictive validity of the P_{ra} instrument among older recipients of managed care. *Journal of the American Geriatrics Society, 45,* 614–617.

Podsiadlo, D., & Richardson, S. (1991). The timed "up and go": A test of basic functional mobility for frail elderly persons. *Journal of the American Geriatrics Society, 39,* 142–148.

Reuben, D. B., Maly, R. C., Hirsch, S. H., Frank, J. C., Oakes, A. M., Siu, A. L., & Hays, R. D. (1997). Physician implementation of and patient adherence to recommendations from comprehensive geriatric assessment. *American Journal of Medicine, 100,* 444–451.

Reuben, D. B., Wolde-Tsadik, G., Pardamean, B., Hammond, B., Borok, G. M., Rubenstein, L. Z., & Beck, J. C. (1992). The use of targeting criteria in hospitalized HMO patients: Results from the demonstration phase of the hospitalized older persons evaluation (HOPE) study. *Journal of the American Geriatrics Society, 40,* 482–488.

Reuben, D. B., Zwanziger, J., Bradley, T. B., Fink, A., Hirsch, S. H., Williams, A. P., Solomon, D. H., & Beck, J. C. (1993). How many physicians will be needed to provide medical care for older persons? Physician manpower needs for the twenty-first century. *Journal of the American Geriatrics Society, 41,* 444–453.

Rich, M. W., Beckham, V., Wittenberg, C., Leven, C. V., Freedland, K. E., & Carney, R. M. (1995). A multidisciplinary intervention to prevent the readmission of elderly patients with congestive heart failure. *New England Journal of Medicine, 333,* 1190–1195.

Rubenstein, L. Z., Bernabei, R., & Wieland, D. (1994). Comprehensive geriatric assessment into the breach. *Aging: Clinical and Experimental Research, 6,* 1–3.

Rubenstein, L. Z., Josephson, K. R., Wieland, D., English, P. A., Sayre, J. A., & Kane, R. L. (1984). Effectiveness of a geriatric evaluation unit: A randomized controlled trial. *New England Journal of Medicine, 311,* 1664–1670.

Rubenstein, L. Z., Stuck, A. E., Siu, A. L., & Wieland, D. (1991). Impacts of geriatric evaluation and management programs on defined outcomes: Overview of the evidence. *Journal of the American Geriatrics Society, 39S,* 8S–16S.

Sager, M. A., Rudberg, M. A., Jalaluddin, M., Franke, T., Inouye, S. K., Landefeld, C. S., Siebens, H., & Winograd, C. H. (1996). Hospital admission risk profile (HARP): Identifying older patients at risk for functional decline following acute medical illness and hospitalization. *Journal of the American Geriatrics Society, 44,* 251–257.

Shah, P. N., Maly, R. C., Frank, J. C., Hirsch, S. H., & Reuben, D. B. (1997). Managing geriatric syndromes: What geriatric assessment teams recommend, what primary care physicians implement, what patients adhere to. *Journal of the American Geriatrics Society, 45,* 413–419.

Solomon, D. H. (1988). Geriatric assessment: Methods for clinical decision-making. *Journal of the American Medical Association, 259,* 2450–2452.

Stuck, A. E., Siu, A. L., Wieland, G. D., & Rubenstein, L. Z. (1993). Comprehensive geriatric assessment: A meta-analysis of controlled trials. *Lancet, 342,* 1032–1036.

Tinetti, M. E., Inouye, S. K., Gill, T. M., & Doucette, J. T. (1995). Shared risk factors for falls, incontinence and functional dependence: Unifying the approach to geriatric syndromes. *Journal of the American Medical Association, 273,* 1348–1353.

Wasson, J., Nelson, G., & Jette, A. (1997). A controlled trial to improve geriatric care in primary care Practices. *Journal of the American Geriatrics Society, 45*(9): S55.

Weinberger, M., Oddonne, E. Z., & Henderson, W. G. (1996). Does increased access to primary care reduce hospital readmissions: Veterans Affairs Cooperative Study Group on primary care and hospital readmission. *New England Journal of Medicine, 334,* 1441–1447.

Weissert, W. G., & Hedrick, S. C. (1994). Lessons learned from research on effects of community-based long-term care. *Journal of the American Geriatrics Society, 42,* 348–353.

Welch, H. G., Wennberg, D. E., & Welch, W. P. (1996). The use of Medicare home health services. *New England Journal of Medicine, 335,* 324–329.

White, J. V., Dwyer, J. T., Posner, B. M., Ham, R. J., & Lipschitz, D. A. (1992). Nutrition screening initiative: Development and implementation of the public awareness checklist and screening tools. *Journal of the American Dietetic Association, 92,* 163–167.

Yesavage, J. A., & Brink, T. L. (1983). Development and validation of a geriatric depression screening scale: A preliminary report. *Journal of Psychiatric Research, 17,* 37–49.

Zimmer, J. G., Groth-Juncker, A., & McCusker, J. (1985). A randomized controlled trial of a home health care team. *American Journal of Public Health, 75,* 134–141.

APPENDIX A P_{ra} Screening Questions

1. In general, would you say your health is:
   - ☐ Excellent
   - ☐ Very good
   - ☐ Good
   - ☐ Fair
   - ☐ Poor

2. In the previous 12 months, have you stayed overnight as a patient in a hospital?
   - ☐ Not at all
   - ☐ One time
   - ☐ Two or three times
   - ☐ More than three times

3. In the previous 12 months, how many times did you visit a physician or clinic?
   - ☐ Not at all
   - ☐ One time
   - ☐ Two or three times
   - ☐ Four to six times
   - ☐ More than six times

4. In the previous 12 months, did you have diabetes?
   - ☐ Yes   ☐ No

5. Have you every had
   A. Coronary heart disease?
   - ☐ Yes   ☐ No   ☐ Don't know

   B. Angina pectoris?
   - ☐ Yes   ☐ No   ☐ Don't know

   C. A myocardial infarction?
   - ☐ Yes   ☐ No   ☐ Don't know

   D. Any other heart attack?
   - ☐ Yes   ☐ No   ☐ Don't know

6. Is there a friend, relative, or neighbor who would take care of you for a few days, if necessary?
   - ☐ Yes   ☐ No   ☐ Don't know

7. Are you
   - ☐ Male   ☐ Female

8. What is your date of birth?

APPENDIX B P_{ra} Scoring Formula

$$P_{ra} = \frac{e^{BX}}{1 + e^{BX}}$$

$BX = -1.802 + .327X_1 + .340X_2 + .552X_3 + .770X_4 + .390X_5 + .545X + .318X_7$
$\quad - .738X_8 + .255X_9 + .327X_{10} + .559X_{11} + .257X_{12} + .319X_{13}$

Predictor variables   0 = absent   1 = present

X_1	very good general health
X_2	good general health
X_3	fair general health
X_4	poor general health
X_5	coronary artery disease
X_6	hospital admission in past year
X_7	>6 physician visits in past year
X_8	no informal caregiver available
X_9	age 75–79 years
X_{10}	age 80–84 years
X_{11}	age 85+ years
X_{12}	male sex
X_{13}	diabetes in past year

APPENDIX C   Components of Comprehensive Assessment

Domain	Topics Often Assessed	Instrument
Personal	Demographics, occupation, education, religion, living situation, finances	
Emotional	Depression	GDS (Yesavage & Brink, 1983)
Functional	Ability to perform ADL, IADL	Katz et al., (1963); OARS, Duke University, 1978
Nutrition	Diet	NSI Checklist, White et al., 1992
Cognition	Cognitive dysfunction	MMSE (Folstein, Folstein, & McHugh, 1975)
Medications	Polypharmacy, nonadherence	
Psychosocial	Relationships, interactions, activities, support	SNS (Lubben, 1988)
Environment	Safety, convenience	
Services	Community and home services used or needed	
Gait	Risk of falls	Up and Go (Podsiadlo & Richardson, 1977)
Preferences	End-of-life care	
Medical history	Conditions, life-style, prevention	CAGE (Mayfield, McLeod, & Hall, 1974)
Physical exam		

GDS = Geriatric Depression Scale; ADL = Activities of Daily Living; IADL = Instrumental Activities of Daily Living; NSI = Nutrition Screening Initiative; MMSE = Mini-Mental State Examination; SNS = Social Network Scale

III

When the Older Person Is Acutely Ill

*T*here is now wide agreement that the hospital provides, for most older patients, an extremely difficult and even hazardous setting. Its propensity to induce confusion is accentuated by its sterile decor and brisk management style. The priorities of the acute care hospital clinicians are, of necessity, directed toward rapid, effective diagnosis and management of severe illnesses or major operative procedures and their associated physiologic challenges. Issues such as prevention of falls, pressure ulcers, protein calorie malnutrition, delirium, and depression often receive far less attention. Most members of the professional staff, well trained in the traditional patterns of inpatient care, have had little training in the special needs of older persons. Many patients, approaching the end of life, are given intensive medical interventions inconsistent with their wishes, and, to date, few effective models have been developed to alter this situation. Finally, the escalating cost of hospital care requires that hospital stays be held to an absolute minimum. As a result, the diagnostic workup is conducted at a rapid pace and is usually accompanied by numerous, frequently invasive tests with little time allowed for the quiet, careful observation that usually provides the best approach to understanding an older person's needs.

The next section describes strategies that are being developed or reexamined in an effort to minimize the problems outlined above and address, more appropriately, the needs of older people who have become acutely ill. Chapter 5 describes how new approaches to medical technology and organization of care are permitting selected patients to be cared for at home. Chapter 6 considers the rapidly expanding role of the hospital emergency department in serving as an interface between community-based care and hospital care. Chapter 7 describes several specific models designed to render the hospital environment more appropriate for older people, addressing, in particular, the losses in cognitive and physical function that often accompany the hospital experience. Chapter 8 describes a new, but fast-growing model, subacute care, which is offering an opportunity for continued medical care in an environment specifically designed to provide interdisciplinary assessment, rehabilitation, and support. Increasingly, this model is also being utilized in the treatment of patients who receive their care through a capitated plan, are facing sudden loss of capacity for maintaining independent life at home, but do not require hospitalization. Chapter 9 addresses the important topic of geriatric rehabilitation, as it occurs in a variety of settings. Chapter 10 emphasizes the need to provide improved levels of palliative care and care for dying patients, whether they are being cared for at home, in the hospital, or some other setting.

A problem with these multiple levels of care is the potential for lack of coordination and sharing of information, as the patient moves through the various sites and programs involved. The need to address this problem through new methods of communication and organization of care is stressed throughout many chapters of this book. This is one of the greatest challenges to our ability to provide effective, comprehensive care for older patients.

5

Care of Acute Illness in the Home

Bruce Leff and John R. Burton

INTRODUCTION

In the last several decades, the hospital has become the standard and pre-eminent venue for the treatment of serious acute illness. It allows physicians to see patients conveniently and efficiently. Patients are closer to sophisticated medical technology and the subspecialist physicians who often direct its use. Although few data demonstrate the hospital's efficacy, and some data suggest otherwise (Slater & Ever-Hadani, 1983), the hospital represents the current paradigm and gold standard of care for serious illness.

In time, however, older patients, some physicians, and many payers have come to recognize that the hospital is not an optimal care environment. Hospital treatment is often uncomfortable and sometimes deprives patients of their dignity and humanity. Iatrogenic complications increase in incidence with patient age (Brennan et al., 1991). Older patients often suffer significant functional decline, which can precipitate a "cascade to dependency" (Creditor, 1993). In addition, evidence increasingly suggests that the culture of care in the acute hospital is often at odds with the wishes of patients (SUPPORT Principal Investigators, 1995). Hospital care has also become extremely expensive.

Because the traditional acute hospital milieu may be harmful to older persons, especially those who are frail, it may make sense to avoid that environment completely. Home Hospital (HH) represents one alternative to hospital acute care. This model brings home to the patient the critical elements of hospital care, medical and nursing care, medicines, and appropriate technology.

HISTORY OF HOME HOSPITAL

HH has been implemented successfully for 30 years, but with few exceptions (Shepperd & Iliffe, 1996) it has received little attention. However, improvements in medical technology in tandem with economic pressures will continue to render HH increasingly feasible. This model demands thoughtful study; economic considerations alone may force its use without proper validation, as health care delivery moves toward capitated models of care.

HH literature is scarce. The best studies occurred in Britain in the 1970s, where randomized controlled trials compared home with hospital treatment for uncomplicated acute myocardial infarction (Hill, Hampton, & Mitchell, 1978; Mather et al., 1976). These studies benefited from examining a discrete, diagnostically crisp illness, generally presumed to require inpatient treatment. They demonstrated that the outcomes of HH treatment were comparable to those of usual hospital care. Recent randomized trials compared hospital with primarily home treatment of proximal deep venous thrombosis; home therapy proved to be feasible, safe, and effective (Koopman et al., 1996; Levine et al., 1996).

DESIGN DIFFICULTIES

The design of the HH and, thus, the designs of studies to evaluate the HH contain inherent difficulties (Leff & Burton, 1996). The design of the HH must first delineate how patients will enter HH care. One model might accept only patients who are on the cusp of being admitted to a hospital from an emergency room or ambulatory site. Another might target patients who are admitted to and clinically stabilized in the acute hospital, expediting their early discharge and treating them at home to complete their hospital care. These two models test different hypotheses and field different interventions. The HH must also decide upon the scope of conditions it will treat. An HH requires more flexibility if it accepts patients with any acute illness than if it accepts only patients with certain diagnoses.

HH patients must be neither so sick that an intensive care setting is required, nor so well that office and/or traditional home care would suffice. Ironically, there are few generally accepted criteria for deciding which patients require hospital admission. Usually, "clinical judgment" prevails, stemming from an uneasy feeling that a patient will be better off in the hospital or needs a service that only the hospital can provide (or can provide with greater convenience), such as intravenous therapy, advanced diagnostic tests, and nursing supervision. Recently, researchers devised a prediction rule to aid in the admission decision by identifying low-risk patients with community-acquired pneumonia (Fine et al., 1997). This classification scheme would deem that many older persons with community-acquired pneumonia, especially those with comorbid illness, require hospital-level care. Unfortunately, such guidelines have not yet undergone the scrutiny of other studies and do not exist for many other common illnesses that result in hospital stays for older persons. Such schemes may not account for social factors, such as caregiver requirements, which are often critical to the decision to hospitalize frail elders.

Obtaining approval for studies to evaluate HH programs may be difficult. Institutional review boards, in the interests of perceived patient safety, may have misgivings about approving randomized controlled trials. In addition, although some data suggest otherwise (Coley et al., 1996), patients may resist HH care because they fear HH is inherently inferior. Also, the families and caregivers may resist because they fear that the HH will shift significant burdens of care or cost to them.

MODELS OF HOME HOSPITAL

Here we will describe two programs of HH, one based in Israel and the other in the United States. The Israeli model (Stessman et al., 1996) provides in-home, physician-supervised, interdisciplinary medical care for patients who would traditionally "require" hospitalization. Patients who require constant medical attention are ineligible for the program. Appropriate patients fall into three care categories: general medical, terminal, and rehabilitative. A senior geriatric physician decides whether to admit each patient within 24 hours of referral to the program. Half the patients come from the acute hospital after having been stabilized there during a truncated stay. The other half come from the community and avoid the inpatient hospital experience entirely. An interdisciplinary team provides the care, with physicians providing 24-hour coverage and home visits as often as needed (a minimum of six visits per month). The average length of stay in HH is 46 days, with 12% of the admissions lasting longer than 90 days. Ten percent of admissions last less than 1 week. The Israeli HH uniquely and appropriately suits Israel's entirely capitated health care delivery system and is now being replicated throughout the country.

Using a quasi-experimental design, a study of the first 741 older patients treated suggested that the Israeli HH decreased rates of hospital utilization and reduced overall costs for the managed care organization that fielded the HH. In addition, results from a limited survey demonstrated high rates of patient satisfaction with the program. The Exra-Mural Hospital in New Brunswick, Canada (Ferguson, 1993) is similar in scope and intent; it appears to be cost-effective (Brown, 1995).

In the U.S., Johns Hopkins is developing a different HH model. The goal of this program is first, to identify appropriate older persons who have certain medical conditions and are on the cusp of admission to the acute hospital, and second, to bring them home to receive their care. The conditions for which a patient may be admitted to HH are community-acquired pneumonia, exacerbation of congestive heart failure, exacerbation of chronic obstructive pulmonary disease, and cellulitis. These conditions, often amenable to treatment at home, account for approximately 20% of the admissions of older persons to the general medical services of acute hospitals.

Recently, the program's criteria for eligibility underwent prospective validation among older adults admitted to a hospital (Leff et al., 1997). Upon admission to the acute hospital, the criteria classified approximately one third of patients as eligible for care in HH. The HH-eligible group experienced, on average, shorter lengths of stay, fewer procedures, fewer complications, and fewer events that could only be handled in the acute hospital setting than those who, by the criteria, were ineligible for HH. Had the criteria of Fine et al (1997) been applied, 83% of the HH-eligible patients with community-acquired pneumonia would have been classified as requiring hospital-level care.

In this HH model, the emergency department or ambulatory care site briefly stabilizes the eligible patient, who is then transported to his or her home in the company of the HH nurse; the HH physician sees the patient within 2 hours. After making a full assessment, the HH physician initiates appropriate diagnostic and therapeutic measures and activates appropriate components of the interdisciplinary care team. The physician visits the patient at home at least daily and is available at all times for urgent or emergency visits to the home. The patient receives direct nursing supervision for the initial portion of his or her stay in HH, the duration of which depends on the level of illness acuity as judged by the physician. The HH nurse also supervises the case management and ensures that the team elements are in place. In addition, HH provides at home diagnostic studies, such as electrocardiograms, radiography, and ultrasound; durable medical equipment; intravenous fluids; intravenous antimicrobials and other medicines; and oxygen and other respiratory therapies. The HH provides diagnostic studies and therapeutics that it cannot provide at home, such as computerized tomography, magnetic resonance imaging, and endoscopy, via brief visits to the appropriate outpatient resource of the acute hospital. A home health agency supplies nurses, aides, therapists, and other ancillary staff to work with the HH in an interdisciplinary fashion. Illness-specific HH "care maps" and clinical outcomes evaluations focus on the medical and functional aspects of care. Communication with the patient's primary care physician has high priority throughout HH care. At the time of discharge from HH, effective communication with the primary care physician and traditional home care providers is especially important to establish, coordinate, and implement appropriate follow-up care. Currently, this model is in the field, undergoing a safety and feasibility trial.

CONCLUSION

With increases in the integration of health care systems, risk sharing, and capitated financing, HH may become increasingly attractive to payers. Rigorous study of HH is critical for several reasons. Continued study will provide information about the appropriate implementation of different HH models, in different locales and care systems. Rigorous research will also determine whether HH clinical outcomes are different from those achieved by hospital care. Finally, differences in outcomes may allow us to improve care provided in acute hospitals.

REFERENCES

Brennan, T. A., Leape, L. L., Laird, N. M., Hebert, L., Localio, A. R., Lawthers, A. G., Newhouse, J. P., Weiler, P. C., & Hiatt, H. H. (1991). Incidence of adverse events and negligence in hospitalized patients: Results of the Harvard Medical Practice Study I. *New England Journal of Medicine, 324,* 370–376.

Brown, M. G. (1995). Cost-effectiveness: The case of home health care physician services in New Brunswick, Canada. *Journal of Ambulatory Care Management, 18,* 13–28.

Coley, C. M., Li, Y. -H., Medsger, A. R., Marrie, T. J., Fine, M. J., Kapoor, W. N., Lave, J. R., Ketsky, A. S., Weinstein, M. C., & Singer, D. E. (1996). Preferences for home vs. hospital care among low-risk patients with community-acquired pneumonia. *Archives of Internal Medicine, 156,* 1565–1571.

Creditor, M. C. (1993). Hazards of hospitalization of the elderly. *Annals of Internal Medicine, 118,* 219–223.

Ferguson, G. (1993). Designed to serve: The New Brunswick Extra-Mural Hospital. *Journal of Ambulatory Care Management, 16,* 40–50.

Fine, M. J., Auble, T. E., Yealy, D. M., Hanusa, B. H., Weissfeld, L. A., Singer, D. E., Coley, C. M., Marrie, T. J., & Kapoor, W. N. (1997). A prediction rule to identify low-risk patients with community-acquired pneumonia. *New England Journal of Medicine, 336,* 243–250.

Fine, M. J., Hough, L. J., Medsger, A. R., Li, Y. -H., Ricci, E. M., Singer, D. E., Marrie, T. J., Coley, C. M., Walsh, M. B., Karpf, M., Lahive, K. C., & Kapoor, W. N. (1997). The hospital admission decision for patients with community-acquired pneumonia. *Archives of Internal Medicine, 157,* 36–44.

Hill, J. D., Hampton, J. R., & Mitchell, R. R. A. (1978). A randomized trial of home-versus-hospital management for patients with suspected myocardial infarction. *Lancet, 1,* 837–841.

Koopman, M. M. W., Prandoni, P., Piovella, F., Ockelford, P. A., Brandjes, D. P. M., Meer, J. v. d., Gallus, A. S., Simonneal, G., Chesterman, C. H., Prins, M. H., Bossuyt, P. M. D., Haes, H. D., Belt, A. G. M. v. d., Sagnard, L., D'Azemar, P., Buller, H. R., & Tasman Study Group. (1996). Treatment of venous thrombosis with intravenous unfractionated heparin administered in the hospital as compared with subcutaneous low-molecular-weight heparin administered at home. *New England Journal of Medicine, 334,* 682–687.

Leff, B., & Burton, J. R. (1996). Acute medical care in the home. *Journal of the American Geriatrics Society, 44,* 603–605.

Leff, B., Burton, L., Bynum, J. W., Harper, M., Greenough, W. B., Steinwachs, D., & Burton, J. R. (1997). Prospective evaluation of clinical criteria to select older persons with acute medical illness for care in a hypothetical home hospital. *Journal of the American Geriatrics Society, 45,* 1066–1073.

Levine, M., Gent, M., Hirsh, J., Leclerc, J., Anderson, D., Weitz, J., Insberg, J., Turpie, A. G., Demers, C., Kovacs, M., Geerts, W., Kassis, J., Desjardins, L., Cusson, J., Cruickshank, M., Powers, P., Brien, W., Haley, S., & Willan, A. (1996). A comparison of low-molecular-weight heparin administered primarily at home with unfractionated heparin administered in the hospital for proximal deep-vein thrombosis. *New England Journal of Medicine, 334,* 677–681.

Mather, H. G., Morgan, D. C., Pearson, N. G., Read, K. L. Q., Shaw, D. B., Steed, G. R., Thorne, M. G., Lawrence, C. J., & Riley, I. S. (1976). Myocardial infarction: A comparison between home and hospital care for patients. *British Medical Journal, 1,* 925–929.

Shepperd, S., & Iliffe, S. (1996). Hospital at home: An uncertain future. *British Medical Journal, 312,* 923–924.

Slater, P., & Ever-Hadani, P. (1983). Mortality in Jerusalem during the 1983 doctors' strike. *Lancet, 2,* 1306.

Stessman, J., Ginsberg, G., Hammerman-Rozenberg, R., Friedman, R., Ronen, D., Israeli, A., & Cohen, A. (1996). Decreased hospital utilization by older adults attributable to a home hospitalization program. *Journal of the American Geriatrics Society, 44,* 591–598.

SUPPORT Principal Investigators. (1995). A controlled trial to improve care for seriously ill hospitalized patients: The study to understand prognoses and preferences for outcomes and risks of treatments (SUPPORT). *Journal of the American Medical Association, 274,* 1591–1598.

6

Older Patients in the Emergency Department

Chris J. Michalakes, Bruce J. Naughton,
Evan Calkins, and Chad Boult

For older persons who are anxious about the apparent seriousness of their illnesses and who are not familiar with emergency processes of care, the emergency department (ED) can be a confusing and frightening place (Baraff et al., 1992). Some view the ED as hostile, uncomfortable, noisy, and threatening to their privacy. Many complain about ineffective communications with ED personnel.

Faced with acute problems superimposed on multiple chronic conditions, emergency physicians must rise to meet complex diagnostic and therapeutic challenges under intense pressure (Wofford, Schwartz, & Byrum, 1993).

Disruptions in care stem from discontinuity between the care provided in the ED and that provided in primary care offices, nursing homes, private homes, and sometimes even hospitals and subacute units. Emergency physicians frequently make crucial clinical decisions without the benefit of even basic information about their older patients' often considerable past and ongoing medical problems, functional limitations, medications, cognitive impairments, social support, or advance directives. Breakdowns in communication about follow-up care may further undermine the effectiveness of emergency care.

Considerable attention has been focused on defining the staffing requirements, operational policies, and architectural arrangements needed to address these inadequacies, and leaders in emergency medicine have recommended that emergency care more meaningfully involve families, friends, and patient advocates. These recommendations have not yet been tested or implemented widely. New systems of care are emerging, but few have been studied systematically. This chapter describes the characteristics of older patients in EDs and some new initiatives designed to improve the emergency care they receive.

OLDER PATIENTS IN THE EMERGENCY DEPARTMENT

Compared with the general older population, older persons who visit EDs are twice as likely to be nonwhite, non–English speaking, and indigent. They often seek emergency care after the failure of self-care for falls or dehydration or after support at home has proven to be inadequate. Depending on the population standard, the location of the ED, and the criteria used for classification, ED physicians report that older ED patients' needs are urgent or emergent in 42% to 81% of cases; one third to one half are admitted to the hospital. Few (2%) regard the ED as their usual source of primary care, but the ED is their most common point of entry into the hospital. Compared with younger patients, ED patients age 65 or older are 4 times more likely to require ambulance transportation, accounting for 36% of all ambulance services and 48% of admissions to coronary care units. Overall, they are 5 to 6 times more likely to be admitted to the hospital or the intensive care unit (Ettinger, Casani, Coon, Muller, & Piazza-Appel, 1987; Lowenstein, Crescenzi, Kern, & Steele, 1986; Strange, Chen, & Sanders, 1992).

SYSTEMS OF EMERGENCY CARE FOR SPECIFIC CONDITIONS

Several recent innovations address older persons' special needs for emergency care. Participating centers have expanded their traditional emergency diagnostic services to include most components of comprehensive geriatric assessment (see chapter 4). Using standardized instruments, nurse clinicians or interdisciplinary teams assess selected older ED patients and make multidimensional recommendations to the ED staff, patients, and their families. Nurse clinicians coordinate, arrange, and sometimes provide follow-up care. Although development and testing of this intervention is incomplete, pilot results have shown that its recipients tend to have fewer subsequent visits to EDs (Gold & Bergman, 1997; Miller, Lewis, Nork, & Morley, 1996).

Cognitive dysfunction complicates the care of 30% to 40% of older ED patients, undermining the reliability of the medical history and the effectiveness of recommendations for post-ED care. In one study, more than one fifth (21.8%) of older ED patients were cognitively impaired, 9% had acutely impaired consciousness, and an additional 10% were delirious. In another study, the ED correctly diagnosed only 17% of delirious or probably delirious seniors and sent many (29%) home still delirious (Lewis, Miller, Morley, Nork, & Lasater, 1995; Naughton, Moran, Kadah, Heman-Ackah, & Longano, 1995).

An interdisciplinary group of emergency health care professionals (the Geriatric Emergency Medicine Task Force) has recommended that all older ED patients be given a brief mental status examination, including questions about short-term recall and orientation to time, place, and person (Sanders, 1995b). Patients unable to answer these questions correctly would then undergo more detailed testing with standardized instruments such as the Mini-Mental Status Examination (Folstein, Folstein, & McHugh, 1975), the Confusion Assessment Method (Inouye, vanDyck, Alessi, Balkin, Siegal, & Horwitz, 1990), or other equivalent tools (Sanders, 1995a). Once diagnosed accurately, older ED patients with cognitive impairment need assistance to compensate for their inabilities to participate fully in their own care. Historical information must be obtained from caregivers and from medical records. Case managers and primary physicians may, in many cases, coordinate and reinforce recommendations for post-ED care.

Other efforts to improve emergency care for older persons have involved developing and testing streamlined systems of care for specific common clinical conditions (e.g., stroke, myocardial infarction, and abuse). For patients with stroke, thrombolytic agents, calcium channel blockers, free radical scavengers, and glutamate antagonists offer new potential to salvage ischemic neurons (Kothari, Barsan, Brott, Broderick, & Ashbrock, 1995). For these pharmaceutical interventions to be effective, however, the patient must receive them within a few hours of the onset of symptoms. Very quickly, emergency personnel must transport the patient to the ED, and the ED personnel must evaluate the clinical situation, perform tests (usually including a brain imaging procedure), consult with a neurologist, discuss treatment options with patients and families, and make therapeutic decisions. To facilitate these processes, stroke teams—which include at least a neurologist, a nurse, a pharmacist, and an imaging technician—are on-call 24 hours a day. Even with these resources in place, however, accomplishing all the needed steps within the 3-hour "window" suggested for effective therapeutic intervention is difficult. Additionally, many older patients have comorbid conditions, making diagnosis more complex, contraindications more likely, and complications more frequent. The definitive role of rapid-response stroke therapies, especially for frail, multiproblem older patients, remains to be determined (Caplan, Mohr, & Kistler, 1997; Grotta, 1997).

Streamlined systems for providing thrombolytic therapy for myocardial infarctions (MIs) face similar challenges. Diagnosis is difficult, treatment is complicated, and mortality is high among older adults. Nevertheless, for those who meet the established eligibility criteria, thrombolytic therapy administered within 6 hours of the onset of symptoms reduces mortality among persons age 75 years or older (American College of Cardiology/ American Heart Association Task Force, 1990). Physicians have difficulty selecting appropriate recipients of emergency intervention for acute MIs, however, offering thrombolytic therapy to only 56% of eligible older patients (Krumholz et al., 1997).

Abuse is another serious problem seen among older adults in the ED. In one study of abuse among older persons who had been hospitalized, 72% were women, 70% were widowed, and 53% lived with a relative. The most common form of abuse (64%) was neglect, such as being left alone for long periods, which had resulted in dehydration, malnutrition, or soiled or inappropriate clothing. Almost half (44%) of the victims had suffered physical abuse, such as beatings, burns, or physical restraint; 40% had been threatened or frightened by their caregivers. Surprisingly, 72% of these patients had not complained of abuse in the ED; review of their hospital records later revealed the causes of their problems (Jones, Dougherty, Schelble, & Cunningham, 1988). Despite growing concerns about elder abuse, systematic approaches to its recognition and treatment in EDs are scarce.

To begin to address some of the present deficits in emergency care for older persons, educational initiatives for emergency physicians are now under way. Supported by a study showing that residency-trained emergency physicians feel inadequately trained in geriatrics (McNamara, Rousseau, & Sanders, 1992), a broad-based task force has recently called for much greater emphasis on geriatric education and research within the discipline of emergency medicine (Sanders, 1995b).

SUMMARY AND CONCLUSIONS

Like hospital care, much of emergency care is technologically sophisticated, but its narrow focus and lack of integration with other venues of health care limits its effectiveness with many older persons. Emergency treatments are increasingly successful in preserving acutely ischemic neural and myocardial tissue, but professionals continue to struggle in their attempts to provide effective care for the complex chronic problems that are most important to their frail older patients.

Looking ahead, leaders in the fields of emergency medicine and geriatrics have articulated nine domains in need of rapid improvement:

- a vision of emergency care as a truly integrated component of a continuum of health care services that includes primary care, home care, nursing home care, hospital care, subacute care, and social services

- education of emergency personnel about the full spectrum of health care needs of older persons
- information systems that would facilitate immediate ED access to current clinical data about older persons, especially those with complicated medical conditions
- smooth, effective transitions for older persons who move between the ED and other sites of health care
- expansion of the ED's scope to include support of the urgent services provided at other sites of care, including patients' homes
- evidence-based guidelines for the application of emergency interventions among older people with comorbid conditions
- definition and integration of the optimal roles of emergency providers in the disciplines of nursing, social work, rehabilitation, and medicine
- systems for measuring and improving the quality of emergency care based on its attainment of the goals of greatest importance to its patients
- reimbursement strategies that reward providers for achieving desirable outcomes more than for providing units of care

As with other venues for care of older persons' acute conditions, the development and testing of innovative care in the ED is still in its infancy.

REFERENCES

American College of Cardiology / American Heart Association Task Force. (1990). ACC/AHA task force report: Guidelines for the early management of patients with acute myocardial infarction. *Journal of the American College of Cardiology, 16,* 249–292.

Baraff, L. J., Bernstein, E., Bradley, K., Franken, C., Gerson, L. W., Hannegan, S. R., Kober, K. S., Lee, S., Marotta, M., & Wolfson, A. B. (1992). Perceptions of emergency care by the elderly: Results of multicenter focus group interviews. *Annals of Emergency Medicine, 21,* 814–818.

Caplan, L. R., Mohr, J. P., & Kistler, J. P. (1997). Should thrombolytic therapy be the first-line treatment for acute ischemic stroke? Thrombolysis—not a panacea for ischemic stroke. *New England Journal of Medicine, 337,* 1309–1310.

Ettinger, W. H., Casani, J. A., Coon, P. J., Muller, D. C., & Piazza-Appel, K. (1987). Patterns of use of the emergency department by elderly patients. *Journal of Gerontology, 42,* 638–642.

Folstein, M. F., Folstein, S. E., & McHugh, P. R. (1975). "Mini-Mental State": A practical method for grading the cognitive status of patients for the clinician. *Journal of Psychiatric Research, 12,* 189–198.

Gold, S., & Bergman, H. (1997). A geriatric consultation team in the emergency department. *Journal of the American Geriatrics Society, 45,* 764–767.

Grotta, J. (1997). Clinical debates: Should thrombolytic therapy be the first-line treatment for acute ischemic stroke? TPA: The current option for most patients. *New England Journal of Medicine, 337,* 1310–1313.

Inouye, S. K., vanDyck, C. H., Alessi, C. A., Balkin, S., Siegal, P., & Horwitz, R. I. (1990). Clarifying confusion: The confusion assessment method—A new method for detection of delirium. *Annals of Internal Medicine, 113,* 941–948.

Jones, J., Dougherty, J., Schelble, D., & Cunningham, W. (1988). Emergency department protocol for the diagnosis and evaluation of geriatric abuse. *Annals of Emergency Medicine, 17,* 1006–1015.

Kothari, R., Barsan, W., Brott, T., Brodrick, J., & Ashbrock, S. (1995). Frequency and accuracy of prehospital diagnosis of acute stroke. *Stroke, 26,* 937–941.

Krumholz, H. M., Murillo, J. E., Chen, J., Vaccarino, V., Radford, M. J., Ellerbeck, E. F., & Wang, Y. (1997). Thrombolytic therapy for eligible elderly patients with acute myocardial infarction. *Journal of the American Medical Association, 277,* 1683–1688.

Lewis, L. M., Miller, D. K., Morley, J. E., Nork, M. J., & Lasater, L. C. (1995). Unrecognized delirium in ED geriatric patients. *American Journal of Emergency Medicine, 13,* 142–145.

Lowenstein, S. R., Crescenzi, C. A., Kern, D. C., & Steel, K. (1986). Care of the elderly in the emergency department. *Annals of Emergency Medicine, 15,* 528–535.

McNamara, R. M., Rousseau, E., & Sanders, A. B. (1992). Geriatric emergency medicine: A survey of practicing emergency physicians. *Annals of Emergency Medicine, 21,* 796–801.

Miller, D. K., Lewis, L. M., Nork, M. J., & Morley, J. E. (1996). Controlled trial of a geriatric case-finding and liaison service in an emergency department. *Journal of the American Geriatrics Society, 44,* 513–520.

Naughton, B. J., Moran, M. B., Kadah, H., Heman-Ackah, Y. & Longano, J. (1995). Delirium and other cognitive impairment in older adults in an emergency department. *Annals of Emergency Medicine, 25,* 751–755.

Sanders, A. B. (1995a). Recognition of cognitive problems in older adults by emergency medicine personnel. *Annals of Emergency Medicine, 25,* 831–833.

Sanders, A. B. (Ed) (1995b). *Emergency care of the elderly person.* St. Louis: Beverly Cracom Publications.

Strange, G. R., Chen, E. H., & Sanders, A. B. (1992). Use of emergency departments by elderly patients: Projections from a multi-center data base. *Annals of Emergency Medicine, 21,* 819–824.

Wofford, J. L., Schwartz, E., & Byrum, J. E. (1993). The role of emergency services in health care for the elderly: A review. *Journal of Emergency Medicine, 11,* 317–326.

7

Care of Older People in the Hospital

Evan Calkins and Bruce J. Naughton

The acute care hospital is a hazardous setting for the care of older patients. Changes that pull older people away from their familiar home environment often threaten their health and well-being (Gillick, Serrell, & Gillick, 1982). The hospital's Spartan decor, high emphasis on technological devices, and rotating personnel create a particularly hostile environment for older people. As pointed out in the introduction to this section, the priorities of most members of the hospital staff center on rapid, effective diagnosis and management of serious acute or intercurrent illness, major operative procedures, and the associated pathophysiologic challenges. Most members of the professional staff are well trained in these components of inpatient care but have had little training in the special needs of older persons. Thus, they tend to overlook issues such as the prevention and treatment of pressure ulcers, protein-calorie malnutrition, falls, and delirium.

In addition to the problem of a strange new environment, the priorities of care inevitably focus on technological interventions, such as respiratory support, parenteral or enterogastric nutrition, and at times cardiopulmonary resuscitation. These measures are appropriate for persons in their middle or later years. For older persons, however, these procedures are often ineffective, inappropriate, or not desired by the patients, their families, or surrogates. Moreover, especially for the older population, these procedures carry high risks. In one study, half of the procedures in older patients that were followed by complications may have been unnecessary in the first place (LeFevre et al., 1992).

Hospital care and the illnesses that precipitate it frequently trigger a cascade of events with serious implications. Hirsch, Sommers, Olsen, Mullen, and Winograd (1990) documented progressive changes in the functional capacity of older persons admitted to the Sanford University Hospital, San Jose, California. Two weeks before admission, 23% were functionally dependent; by discharge, 41% were dependent. Even people who previously functioned independently at home often suffer losses of functional capacity during hospitalization, such that they must accept permanent residence in a long-term care or assisted living facility upon discharge (Creditor 1993; Mor, Wilcox, Rakowski, & Hiris, 1994). For some people, this cascade of events leads to death. By 6 months after hospital admission, mortality for persons age 75 or older is more than 20% (Fretwell et al., 1990). Another study observed that 25% of hospitalized patients age 65 or older had died within 12 months of admission (Reuben et al., 1995).

In this chapter, we summarize factors that have been shown to predispose to these losses. We then detail four systems designed to enhance the outcomes of older patients in the hospital setting, all of which have been evaluated in randomized clinical trials. We conclude by enumerating topics that deserve increased attention in the future.

ANTECEDENTS OF DECLINE IN THE HOSPITAL

Age is not the only, nor even the most important, predictor of adverse outcomes of hospitalization. Table 7.1, summarizes characteristics that predict unfavorable outcomes. Advancing age, impaired functional status before admission, and the presence of dementia or delirium most consistently predict prolonged hospital stay, functional decline, increased frequency of complications or iatrogenic events, the inability to be discharged home, and death.

Two teams of investigators have designed systems for quantifying the risk of adverse outcomes by combining several of these factors. Researchers at Yale University studied a cohort of 193 patients, age 75 years or older, admitted to a teaching hospital (Inouye et al., 1993). They classified each patient's risk level according to selected risk factors for functional decline (pressure ulcers, cognitive impairment, functional impairment, and low social activity level). The likelihood of discharge to a nursing home ranged from 4% for the low-risk group (no risk factors) to 22% for the high-risk group (three or four risk factors). The likelihood of death increased from 2% for the low-risk group to 19% for the high-risk group.

Sager and colleagues (1996) developed another scoring system, the Hospital Admission Risk Profile (HARP). Previous research had shown that three pre-admission variables—advanced age, reduced cognitive function, and independence in any of the six instrumental activities of daily living—predict subsequent loss of functional capacity (Lawton & Brody, 1969). These investigators assigned each factor a weight, depending on the extent to which it predicted functional decline. They found that the summary score for all three factors at admission correlated closely with functional decline both during hospitalization and at reassessment 3 months after discharge.

SYSTEMS OF IN-HOSPITAL CARE

The Geriatric Evaluation and Management (GEM) Unit

The first randomized controlled study of a system designed to address the issues cited above evaluated an inpatient GEM unit of a Veterans Administration hospital—15 beds within the hospital's intermediate care area (Rubenstein et al., 1984). Staff members included an attending geriatrician, a geriatrics fellow, a physicians' assistant, a social worker, nurses, and nursing assistants, and other professionals. The staff maintained direct, as opposed to consultative, responsibility for all aspects of patient care.

Researchers enrolled appropriate patients into a study of this unit 1 week after admission to the acute areas of the hospital. GEM staff made particular efforts to identify patients who were likely to benefit from the intervention. Candidates were age 65 or older and had persistent medical, functional, or psychological problems that were likely to interfere with discharge. The final sample, 123 patients, represented only 8.5% of all patients screened for the study. Following enrollment, the patients were randomly assigned either to the GEM unit or to a control group that received usual care. GEM patients spent an average of 18 days in acute care and 80 days in intermediate care, for a total of 98 days; control patients spent 34 days in acute care and 28 days in intermediate care, for a total of 62 days. After discharge, the intervention patients received follow-up care in the hospital's geriatric clinic, while the controls attended the general medical clinics.

At discharge, the two groups differed substantially in posthospital place of residence: 73% of the study patients and 53% of the controls were able to return home or to a board-and-care facility. The percentage who died in the hospital was almost identical for both groups. However, during the following year the percentage of deaths was significantly lower among the study patients (23.8% vs. 48.3%). The authors estimated that the cost of care for the GEM patients, including that on the GEM unit and during follow-up in the geriatric clinic, "was more than recouped over the course of the 12 month follow-up period by savings in the use of other services, such as acute hospitalization and nursing home care." (Rubenstein et al., 1994, p. 1669).

This study is still a classic demonstration that comprehensive interdisciplinary care can improve the outcomes of hospital care, but the application

TABLE 7.1 Characteristics Found to be Associated With Adverse

Risk Factor	Criteria	Frequency
Age		
Impaired function	Independence in fewer than 6 IADLS[a,2]	66%[1]–76%[2]
Decreased cognitive function	<20 on Mini-Mental Status Exam[b] or 0–14 on 21-item version of MMSE[2]	40%[2]
Delirium	Confusion Assessment Method[c]	17%–29%[1,4,6]
Depression	Geriatric Depression Scale[d]	45%[12]
Protein-calorie malnutrition	Subnormal in 3 of 5 variables[9]	20%[9]
Pressure ulcers	Skin breakdown (Grades I–IV) at any of 11 pressure points	11%[1]
Pre-admission falls	Any during the 3 months before admission[3]	6%[4]
Pre-illness decrease in social activity	3 or fewer of 11 social functions in typical month	+[1*]
Socioeconomic problems	Living alone—elder abuse[3]	26%[3]
Prolonged bed rest	Majority of time in bed during 2 weeks before admission	
Incontinence		27%[3,4]
Polypharmacy	5 or more prescription drugs	42%[2,3]
Physical illness	APACHEII	14%[1]
Multiple organ disease[9]		
Previous residence in a nursing home		
Hearing impairment		
Vision impairment	Verbal report[3]	16%[3]

The criteria cited represent one example of the characteristics studied by various investigators. The numbers refer to publications containing the information. The full reference is listed alphabetically in the bibliography. The asterisk, associated with references 1 and 2, refers to the fact that the four variables were assessed in a composite fashion, rather than individually. *Sources:* (1) Inouye, Wagner, Acampora, Horwitz (1993), (2) Sager, Redberg, Jalaluddin, et al. (1996), (3) Satish, Winograd, Chavez, et al. (1996), (4) Gillick, Serrell, & Gillick (1982), (5) Hirsch, Sommers, Olsen, et al. (1990), (6) O'Keefe, & Lavan (1997), (7) Francis, Martin, & Kapora (1990), (8) Winograd, Gerity, Chung, et al. (1991), (9) Cederholm, Jagren, & Hellstrom (1995), (10) Cole (1993), (11) Levkoff, Evans, Liptzin, et al. (1992), (12) Kitchell, Veith, Okimoto, & Raskine (1982), (13) LeFevre, Feinglass, Potts, et al. (1992), (14) Jahnigen, Hannon, Laxson, & Laforce (1982), (15) Koenig, Shelp, Goli, et al. (1989). *Methodology:* (a) Lawton & Brody, (1969), (b) Folstein, Folstein, & McHugh, (1975), (c) Inouye et al., (1900), (d) Yesavage & Brink, (1983).

Outcomes for Older Patients Admitted to Acute Care Hospitals

		Adverse Outcomes		
Mortality During Hospitalization	Length of Stay	Complications (Infectious or Iatrogenic Events)	Decline in Function During Hospitalization	Placement in Nursing Home at Discharge
+[2]	+[5]	+[13,14]	+[2,3,8]	+[2]
+[3]	+[3,5]	+[13]	+[2,3,8]	+[3]
+[1*]	+[2]	+[13]	+[1,1*,2,3,4,8]	+[1*,2]
+[10,11]	+[6,7,10]	+[6]	+[3,6]	+[3,6,7,10]
			+[3]	
+[9]	+[9]	+[9]		
+[1*]			+[1*,4,8]	+[1*]
			+[8]	
			+[1*]	+[1*]
		+[3]		
			+[3]	
			+[3]	
		+[14]	+[3]	+[3]
			+[14]	
+[9]	+[9]			
			+[1]	
			+[3]	
			+[3]	+[3]

of these findings to the modern health care system is limited. The study took place in a heavily staffed government-run and -financed facility that provided extended hospitalization, circumstances that are no longer possible. Candidates, carefully selected for high likelihood of benefit, included only 8.5% of those screened. It is also difficult to desegregate the benefits of the GEM unit from those of the follow-up ambulatory care in a geriatric outpatient clinic.

Six years passed before a comparable randomized control study was undertaken in a community-based facility (Applegate et al., 1990). These patients, age 65 or older, were admitted to the acute care services of a rehabilitative hospital and appeared to be at high risk for nursing home placement. They were randomly assigned to the control group ($n = 77$) or to the Geriatric Assessment Unit ($n = 78$) following stabilization of their acute problems. The care on the Assessment Unit was similar to that provided on the aforementioned GEM unit: The unit staff provided all care. When patients reached their rehabilitative goals or a stable level of function, they were discharged to the care of personal physicians without further involvement by the Geriatric Assessment Unit team. Control patients received usual care.

The mean length of stay in the unit was 24 days. By 6 weeks following discharge, only 8% of patients assigned to the Geriatric Assessment Unit were living in institutions, as compared with 24% of controls; by 6 months, these values were 11% and 26%, respectively. Six months following discharge, the intervention group had significantly greater functional improvement than the controls, but these differences dissipated over the next 6 months. Improved outcomes also included mortality: Six months after randomization, 10% of the patients in the intervention group had died, as compared with 21% of those in the control group. These differences also became less significant at 1 year. The fact that, following discharge from the program, all patients received ambulatory or nursing home care under direction of their private physicians, rather than through members of the geriatric care team, suggests that the benefits, described, were achieved by virtue of the relatively brief hospitalization in the Geriatric Assessment Unit, a somewhat surprising but impressive conclusion.

The Acute Care for the Elderly (ACE) Unit

Both of the studies described above examined the effectiveness of comprehensive care *following* a period of hospitalization on acute medical wards. Unfortunately, the most significant declines in functional and cognitive capacity often occur during the initial days of hospital care (Hirsch et al., 1990). Building on the observation that it is easier to prevent functional losses than it is to restore them, geriatricians have recently attempted to improve the acute phase of hospital care.

Investigators at The Case Western Reserve University Hospital identified 651 patients upon admission who were age 70 or older and did not require intensive care (Landefeld, Palmer, Kresevic, Fortinsky, & Kowal, 1995). They randomly assigned half of the patients to the Acute Care for the Elderly (ACE) unit and half to traditional ward services. No effort was made to limit admission to patients who were deemed to have the highest likelihood of benefitting from the program. All patients received care from internal medicine attending physicians and residents who worked on both the intervention and control units. Care on the control units followed conventional patterns. On the ACE units, a geriatrician and a geriatric nurse practitioner provided detailed and continuous on the spot supervision, and nurses, aides, rehabilitation therapists, social workers, a pharmacist, and a dietitian functioned as an interdisciplinary team with a rehabilitative orientation.

A primary nurse assigned to each patient assessed, daily, each patient's physical, cognitive, and psychosocial function and implemented established protocols designed to improve self-care, competence, nutrition, mobility, sleep, skin care, mood, and cognition and to minimize the adverse effects of procedures, such as urinary catherization. The social worker coordinated discharge planning from the day of admission. The whole team conducted daily rounds led by the medical and nursing directors, and made recommendations to the attending physicians. Additionally, the hospital modified the physical environment of the ACE unit by maintaining uncluttered hallways, displaying large clocks and calendars, and installing carpeting, handrails, door levers, and elevated toilet seats. The entire operation was coordinated and tightly administered by a senior nurse, who had committed herself to the success of the program over the course of several years, and whose personality suited her for this commanding role

Results: Of patients in the ACE group, 21% improved their capacity to perform basic activities of daily living by the time of discharge, a significantly greater proportion than the 13% of patients in the control group who improved these capacities. Forty-three percent of ACE patients were discharged to a long-term care facility, as compared with 60% of the control group. The groups did not differ significantly in mortality or length of stay. Even allowing for the architectural and special staffing costs of the ACE unit, the costs of care for the patients in the two groups were similar (Covinski et al., 1997).

The geriatric team did not make special arrangements to follow up their patients after discharge. Three months after discharge, the two groups of patients did not differ significantly in their function status or in the proportion who were readmitted to acute care hospitals (34% for the ACE group and 36% for the control group). This study illustrates that protocol-driven, function-oriented interdisciplinary interventions, introduced early in the hospital care of older patients, facilitates functional recovery and return to home. Without continued follow up by the geriatric group, however, these benefits were soon lost.

Geriatric Consultation

While the geographically defined, team care–oriented ACE unit appears to be an excellent model for the acute phase of inpatient geriatric care, the sheer number of older patients, many of whom are frail and at high risk for losing function, exceeds the present capacity of many hospitals to accommodate them in ACE units. Can other models of care adequately address the needs of older patients on general "undifferentiated" wards? The approach to this problem that has received the greatest attention is the use of interdisciplinary geriatric consultation teams. Reports from more than a dozen well-designed, randomized controlled studies of this intervention have been published.

An early model provided encouragement regarding the effectiveness of this approach (Barker et al., 1985). The authors described how communitywide implementation of geriatric consultation alleviated the "backup" of difficult-to-discharge older patients in alternate level of care (ALC) wards of acute care hospitals. All participating hospitals showed significant decreases in the number of ALC patients, an outcome not shared by nonparticipating hospitals in the same community.

Unfortunately, with only a few exceptions, subsequent studies of inpatient consultation have shown little benefit in terms of patient survival, functional capacity, duration of hospitalization, or likelihood of returning home. In one randomized trial, investigators targeted older inpatients at four HMO hospitals who were at risk for adverse outcomes (Reuben et al., 1995). The results showed no significant differences between intervention and control groups in terms of physical or cognitive function or survival rates, during either the hospital stay or the following 12 months.

Another randomized study of a Veterans Administration hospital included older men hospitalized on the medical, surgical, and psychiatric services (McVey, Becker, Saltz, Feussner, & Cohen, 1989). All received an initial evaluation by an interdisciplinary geriatric team, composed of a geriatrician, a geriatric fellow, a geriatric clinic nurse specialist, and a social worker. For the patients in the intervention group, the team recorded its evaluation and recommendations in the charts, communicated personally with the provider staff, and followed the patients regularly. For the patients in the control group, the team simply inserted a problem list in each chart. At the time of discharge, overall functional capacity did not differ significantly between the two groups.

A similar study, undertaken at a general hospital in Halifax, Nova Scotia, showed that, at the time of discharge, the intervention and control groups did not differ significantly with regard to mortality, mean length of hospital stay, proportion discharged to a nursing home, functional capacity, or mental status (Hogan & Fox, 1990). After discharge, however, the two groups received quite different care. The control group received traditional follow-up care. The intervention patients received written or telephone contact, follow-up care in the geriatric outpatient clinic, or a home visit by the consulting physician, who sent recommendations to the patient's primary physician. Evaluation at 180 days following discharge showed significantly enhanced survival among the intervention group. One year after discharge, the difference in survival was no longer apparent, but the intervention patients had achieved a statistically significant improvement in functional capacity compared with the controls. The improved longer-term follow-up results may be more attributable to the pattern of follow-up care than to the consultations conducted during the hospital stay.

In summary, most studies have failed to show that inpatient geriatrics consultation produces significant improvements in functional capacity, mortality, duration of stay, or future placement of the patients involved (Stuck, Siu, Wieland, Adams, & Reubenstein, 1993). In considering possible explanations for this generally negative result, the different authors offered several possibilities. One was the less-than-optimal targeting of candidates for the intervention. Reuben et al. (1995) pointed out that the criteria for entry into their study may have included a number of patients whose function was sufficiently limited that the potential for improvement was minimal. Additional possible explanations, cited by the authors, included the high quality of care given to the patients in the control group by the HMO physicians, many of whom had received some training in geriatrics in continuing education programs, and the fact that the same primary care physicians cared for patients both in the intervention and control groups.

It seems more likely to us that the explanation was one offered by McVey et al. (1985) for the failure of success in their program. "In our study," they state, "although recommendations were complied with in a high proportion of the cases, this fact simply assured that some attention was paid to the problem but did not assure the depth of the quality of service delivery as conceived by the team. A recommendation . . . did not necessarily mean that the actual care was delivered in exactly the same manner desired." (McVey et al., 1985, pp. 83–84). They go on to point out that the typical consultation, offered by a specialty group, requires or recommends a very simple limited response, generally of a procedural nature—an additional test or specific intervention. A geriatric consultation, by contrast, requires, also, a *behavioral* change on the part of the provider. The issue is not so much what is done, but *how* it is done. As has been demonstrated abundantly, behavior changes are difficult to achieve. There is increasing agreement that this is why effective interventions in geriatric care, whether in the setting of a hospital, clinic or patient's home, are almost always dependent on the direct efforts of providers especially interested in and skilled in the multifaceted characteristics and needs of older persons.

Nurse-Based Comprehensive Assessment and Care

Researchers at Yale University initiated an entirely different approach to improving hospital care of frail older persons, an approach that acknowledged the nursing staff's vital contributions (Inouye et al., 1993). The study involved five acute noninvasive medical units, two randomly selected as intervention sites and three as controls. Regularly assigned house staff and attending physicians provided the medical care on all units.

Each experimental unit had several geriatric resource nurses, staff nurses who exhibited interest in the care of frail older patients and had received special training in the identification and management of older people at risk for functional decline during hospitalization. A gerontologic nurse specialist trained and supervised the geriatric resource nurses, identified patients who were appropriate candidates for intensive gerontologic nursing care, surveyed these patients daily, conducted twice-weekly gerontologic nursing rounds, and coordinated twice-weekly interdisciplinary team conferences. Issues receiving special attention included maintenance of activities of daily living, nutrition, incontinence, delirium, dementia, and falls. The nursing staff made specific recommendations to the medical house staff and attending physicians. A geriatrician provided medical and gerontologic consultations to the nurses upon their request. The geriatrician also maintained physician-to-physician communication with consulting specialists and provided lectures and seminars on request. Comparison of matched (nonrandomized) patients revealed that fewer of the patients on the intervention units than on the control units exhibited functional decline (41% vs. 64%). The authors did not provide data on mortality and number of patients discharged home.

Both the nurse-based model at Yale University and the ACE unit at Case Western Reserve University were established institutions with strong schools of nursing that have a special interest in gerontology, and both have strong programs in geriatric medicine as well. Both models hold potential for decreasing functional loss in hospitalized, frail older patients and deserve wider study.

LESSONS LEARNED FROM THE EVIDENCE CITED

Traditionally, hospitals have provided a difficult and challenging environment for older patients. Hospitals of the future may be able to effect better outcomes by incorporating four principles from these studies into their systems of care:

1. early identification of older patients who are at greatest risk
2. comprehensive assessment of physical, cognitive, and social functioning conducted by the same professionals who will provide ongoing care
3. team-orientated care, using predetermined and validated protocols for addressing specific gerontologic conditions
4. integration of hospital care with community-based follow-up care

REFERENCES

Applegate, W. B., Miller, S. T., Graney, M. J., Elan, J. T., Burns, R., & Akins, D. E. (1990). A randomized controlled trial in a geriatric assessment unit in a community rehabilitation hospital. *New England Journal of Medicine, 322*, 1572–1578.

Barker, W. H., Williams, T. F., Zimmer, J. G., vanBuren, C., Vincent, S. J., & Pickrel, M. S. (1985). Geriatric consultation teams in acute hospitals. Impact on back-up of elderly patients. *Journal of the American Geriatrics Society, 33*, 422–428.

Cederholm, T., Jagren, C., & Hellstrom, K. (1995). Outcome of protein-energy malnutrition in elderly medical patients. *American Journal of Medicine, 98*, 67–74.

Cole, M. G., & Primeau, F. J. (1993). Prognosis of delirium in elderly hospitalized patients. *Canadian Medical Association Journal, 149*, 41–46.

Covinski, K. E., King, J. T., Quinn, L. M., Siddique, R., Palmer, R., Kresevic, D. M., Fortinsky, R. H., Kowal, J. & Landefeld, C. S. (1997). Do Acute Care for Elders units increase hospital costs? A cost analysis using the hospital perspective. *Journal of the American Geriatrics Society, 45*, 729–734.

Creditor, M. D. (1993). Hazards of hospitalization in the elderly. *Journal of the American College of Physicians, 118*, 219–223.

Folstein, M. F., Folstein, S. E., McHugh, P. R. (1975). "Mini-mental state"; A practical method for grading the cognitive state of patients for the clinician. *Journal of Psychiatric Research, 12*, 189–198.

Frances, J., Martin, D., & Kapoor, W. N. (1990). A prospective study of delirium in hospitalized elderly. *Journal of the American Medical Association, 263*, 1097–1101.

Fretwell, M. D., Raymond, P. M., McGarvey, S. T., Owens, N., Traines, M., Silliman, R. A., & Mor, V. (1990). The senior care study: A controlled trial of a consultative-unit-based geriatric assessment program in acute care. *Journal of the American Geriatrics Society, 38*, 1073–1081.

Gillick, M. R., Serrell, N. A., & Gillick, L. S. (1982). Adverse consequences of hospitalization in the elderly. *Social Science Medicine, 16*, 1003–1038.

Hirsch, C. H., Sommers, L., Olsen, A., Mullen, L., & Winograd, C. H. (1990). The natural history of functional mobility in hospitalized older patients. *Journal of the American Geriatrics Society, 38,* 1296–1303.

Hogan, D. B., & Fox, R. A. (1990). A prospective controlled trial of a geriatric consultation team in an acute care hospital. *Age and Ageing, 19,* 107–113.

Inouye, S. K., Acampora, D., Miller, R. L., Fulmer, T., Hurst, L. D., & Cooney, L. M., Jr. (1993). The Yale Geriatric Care Program: A model of care to prevent functional decline in hospitalized elderly patients. *Journal of the American Geriatrics Society, 41,* 1345–1352.

Inouye, S. K., Wagner, D. R., Acampora, D., Horwitz, R. I., Cooney, L. M., Jr., Hurst, L. D., & Tinetti, M. E. (1993). A predictive index for functional decline in hospitalized elderly medical patients. *Journal of General Internal Medicine, 8,* 645–652.

Inouye, S. K., van Dyck, C. H., Alessi, C. A., Balkin, S., Siegal, A. P., & Horwitz, R. I. (1990). Clarifying confusion: The Confusion Assessment Method; a new method for Detection of Delirium. *Annals of Internal Medicine, 113,* 941–948.

Jahnigen, D., Hannon, C., Laxson, L., & LaForce, F. M. (1982). Iatrogenic disease in hospitalized elderly veterans. *Journal of the American Geriatric Society, 30,* 387–390.

Kitchell, M. A., Barnes, R. F., Veith, R. C., Okimoto, J. T., & Raskind, M. A. (1982). Screening for depression in hospitalized geriatric medical patients. *Journal of the American Geriatrics Society, 30,* 174–177.

Koenig, H. G., Shelp, F., Goli, V., Cohen, H. J., & Blazer, D. G. (1989). Survival and health care utilization in elderly medical inpatients with major depression. *Journal of the American Geriatrics Society, 37,* 599–606.

Landefeld, C. S., Palmer, R. M., Kresevic, D. M., Fortinsky, R. H., & Kowal, J. (1995). A randomized trial of care in a hospital medical unit especially designed to improve the functional outcomes of acutely ill older patients. *New England Journal of Medicine, 332,* 1338–1344.

Lawton, M. P., & Brody, E. M. (1969). Assessment of older people: Self-maintaining and instrumental activities of daily living. *Gerontologist, 9,* 179–186.

LeFevre, S., Feinglass, J., Potts, S., Soglin, L., Yarnold, P., Martin, G., & Webster, J. R. (1992). Iatrogenic complications in high-risk elderly patients. *Archives of Internal Medicine, 152,* 2074–2080.

Levkoff, S. E., Evans, D. A., Liptzin, B., Cleary, P. D., Lipsitz, L. A., Wettle, T., Reilly, C. H., Pilgrim, D. M., Shor, J., & Rowe, J. (1992). Delirium: The occurrence and persistence of symptoms among elderly hospitalized patients. *Archives of Internal Medicine, 152,* 334–340.

McVey, L. J., Becker, P. M., Saltz, C. C., Feussner, J. R., & Cohen, H. D. (1989). Effect of a geriatric consultation team on functional status of elderly hospitalized patients: A randomized controlled clinical trial. *Annals of Internal Medicine, 110,* 79–84.

Mor, V., Wilcox, V., Rakowski, W., & Hiris, J. (1994). Functional transitions among the elderly: Patterns, predictors and related hospital use. *American Journal of Public Health, 84,* 1274–1280.

O'Keefe, S., & Lavan, J. (1997). The prognostic significance of delirium in older hospital patients. *Journal of the American Geriatrics Society, 45,* 174–178.

Reuben, D. B., Borok, G. M., Wolde-Tsadik, G., Ershoff, D. H., Fishman, L. K., Ambrosini, V. L., Liu, Y., Rubenstein, L. Z., & Beck, J. C. (1995). A randomized trial of comprehensive geriatric assessment in the care of hospitalized patients. *New England Journal of Medicine, 332,* 1345–1350.

Rubenstein, L. Z., Josephson, K. R., Wieland, G. D., English, P. A., Sayre, J. A., & Kane, R. L. (1984). Effectiveness of a geriatric evaluation unit: A randomized clinical trial. *New England Journal of Medicine, 311,* 1664–1670.

Sager, M. A., Rudberg, M. A., Jalaluddin, M., Franke, T., Inouye, S. K., Landefeld, C. S., Siebens, H., & Winograd, C. H. (1996). Hospital Admission Risk Profile (HARP): Identifying older patients at risk for functional decline following acute medical illness and hospitalization. *Journal of the American Geriatrics Society, 44,* 251–257.

Satish, S., Winograd, C. H., Chavez, C., & Bloch, D.A. (1996). Geriatric targeting criteria as predictors of survival and health care utilization. *Journal of the American Geriatrics Society, 44,* 914–921.

Stuck, W. E., Siu, A. L., Wieland, G. D., Adams, T., & Reubenstein, L. Z. (1993). Comprehensive geriatric assessment: A meta-analysis controlled trial. *Lancet, 342,* 1032–1036.

Winograd, C. H., Gerety, M. B., Chung, M., Goldstein, M. K., Dominquez, F. J., & Vollone, R. (1991). Screening for frailty: Criteria and predictors of outcomes. *Journal of the American Geriatrics Society, 39,* 778–784.

Yesavage, J. A., & Brink, T. L. (1982–1983). Development and validation of a geriatric depression screening scale: A preliminary report. *Journal of Psychiatric Research, 17,* 37–49.

8

Subacute Care

Thomas vonSternberg, Karen Connors,
and Evan Calkins

In the past five years, one of the most dramatic changes in the system of care for older people has been the emergence and exponential growth of subacute care. Also called transitional care, subacute care was originally designed to provide intermediary services between acute hospital care and the patient's return to home, a nursing home, or a supportive residence. In this chapter, we define subacute care, describe several models, and review two studies that compared outcomes of subacute care with those achieved by traditional rehabilitation programs. Finally, the chapter will present results from one particularly successful subacute unit to illustrate the potential inherent in this pattern of care.

The Medicare Prospective Payment System, which began in the mid-1980s, created direct incentives for hospitals to shorten lengths of stay; this became the initial impetus for the development of subacute care (Morrisey, Sloan, & Valvona, 1988). Many hospitalized older patients who no longer require high-technology or intensive treatment still need ongoing medical or rehabilitative attention more continuously than home or office care can provide. (For example, older patients undergoing coronary artery bypass grafts, aggressive chemotherapy, complex orthopedic and vascular procedures, and infectious disease therapy—procedures that accord them major convalescence and rehabilitation needs.) As chapter 7 attests, hospitalization of older people for any reason is almost accompanied by rapid losses of functional capacity, which usually persist after the anticipated and allowable period of acute hospitalization and require ongoing medical as well as rehabilitative therapy. It is in this context that the concept of subacute care had its genesis. Managed care, with its incentives to provide appropriate care efficiently, uses subacute care to facilitate earlier discharge of patients from the acute hospital.

DESCRIPTION OF SUBACUTE CARE MODELS

The Joint Commission on Accreditation of Health Care Organizations (JCAHO) developed a definition for subacute care that has been widely accepted:

> Sub-acute care is comprehensive inpatient care designed for someone who has an acute illness, injury, or exacerbation of a disease process. It is goal-oriented treatment rendered immediately after, or instead of, acute hospitalization to treat one or more specific active complex medical conditions or to administer one or more technically complex treatments, in a context of a person's underlying long term conditions and overall situation. Generally, the individual's condition is such that the care does not depend heavily on high-technology monitoring or complex diagnosis procedures. Sub-acute care requires the coordinated services of an interdisciplinary team, including physicians, nurses, and other relevant professional disciplines, who are trained and knowledgeable. ("Accreditation protocol for subacute programs" 1996, pp. 2–3).

The policy and procedure requirements of a subacute unit depend on the unit's location (e.g., in a section of an acute care hospital or in a skilled nursing home) and whether the unit desires JCAHO accreditation. For the subacute unit located in an acute care hospital, the policies must conform to those of the hospital. A unit in a nursing home must conform to that facility's regulatory and JCAHO requirements, if it desires JCAHO accreditation. Accreditation provides the unit a "stamp of approval," ensuring an appropriate level of staffing and quality of care.

Each unit must include a minimum of 15 beds located within a geographically defined area. Subacute patients may not be dispersed among long-term residents. The ratio of nurses to patients should exceed that of a typical long-term care facility, and the nursing staff should have acute hospital experience. Registered nurses should be available during all shifts, supplemented by a well-trained licensed practical nursing staff (vonSternberg et al., 1997). Units that accept admissions during evenings and weekends must provide full staff 24 hours a day, 7 days a week.

Nurse practitioners (NPs) contribute substantially to the operation of many subacute units. In addition to providing advice and assistance to the nursing staff, NPs play an important role in reassessing patients when they have a change of clinical status and in helping with admissions evaluations, which (for JCAHO approval) must be completed within 48 hours of admission. The physician must review and cosign these evaluations, and the facility needs to accept a practice agreement between the physician and the NP.

The unit should have a designated physician, often a geriatrician. In addition to understanding the rehabilitative needs of older patients, a geriatrician is well suited to manage complex medical problems, together with such issues as advance directives, depression, polypharmacy, and quality assurance (Ouslander, Osterweil, & Morley, 1997). The designated physician usually provides ongoing medical care in the context of an interdisciplinary team. Contacts with primary care physicians or specialists can be arranged through outpatient visits. Physicians typically see patients in subacute units at least twice a week and bill Medicare based on appropriately documented effort and complexity.

Since the subacute unit provides both medical care and rehabilitation, it includes appropriate rehabilitation staff to provide intensive speech, physical, and occupational therapy. Many subacute units also provide recreational therapy. The unit may employ the rehabilitation staff, or it may obtain their services on a contractual basis. Depending on the focus of the units, nurses may administer intravenous antibiotics, administer oxygen and monitor blood gases, administer respiratory therapy, obtain same-day laboratory results, manage components of renal dialysis, and administer intramuscular or intravenous pain management. Discharge planning from subacute care is as important and complex as that from a hospital. Ideally, the social worker or case manager assigned to this task is a full-time member of the unit's staff.

Team efforts are coordinated through interdisciplinary conferences that include the designated physician, an NP, registered nurses, a social worker, a dietitian, and rehabilitation therapists. The team reviews the progress of all patients and plans the care of new admissions. Candidates especially appropriate for admission include patients who have undergone hip and knee replacements, have fractured a hip, have suffered a stroke, have become deconditioned while recovering from surgery or acute illness, have existing functional deficits, or require complex therapies that cannot be provided at home.

STAFFING AND SERVICES

Subacute units share with the traditional rehabilitation units the goal of restoring physical function to older patients who have become deconditioned following a period of acute care in a hospital. Both entities may be located within acute care hospitals or in alternative community settings. Staffs of both types of units rely on the concepts of interdisciplinary team care, and they address psychosocial as well as physical function. However, there are significant differences. The major goal of a rehabilitation department is to restore physical function. The medical director must be a certified physiatrist. To qualify for admission, a patient must have sufficient stamina and strength to spend 3 hours a day in intensive physical, occupational, or speech therapy, or a combination thereof.

Admission to a subacute unit implies an expectation that an orchestrated comprehensive program of assessment, care, and rehabilitation will enable the patient to return home or to a less intensive environment within a short period of time, usually up to 3 weeks. Most patients have multiple, chronic medical and/or psychiatric disorders, as well as functional impairments. The intensity of the various therapies, including medical management, are customized in accordance with the patient's particular needs. While a physiatrist may function as the designated physician for a subacute unit, the role is most often performed by an internist or family physician, ideally one with experience in geriatrics. A physiatrist may or may not be on staff as a consultant. In addition, major responsibilities are usually assigned to an NP, ideally a gerontological NP (GNP). Thus, subacute units provide a more varied pattern of assessment and care than that provided by rehabilitation departments. Usually, the cost of care in a subacute unit is substantially lower than that of an acute care hospital or rehabilitation unit, but somewhat higher than that of a traditional skilled nursing facility.

DIRECT ADMISSION FROM HOME TO A SUBACUTE UNIT

With increasing experience with subacute care's effective combination of medical and rehabilitative care, physicians and administrators have begun to ask whether these units could play a comparable role in meeting the immediate needs of community-dwelling older people for whom relatively minor acute illness or progressive loss of physical function threatens the ability to remain home. Health care providers who work under Medicare risk contracts can admit patients directly to subacute units in skilled nursing facilities without the otherwise mandatory 3-day period of previous hospitalization. Although data on the effectiveness of this approach is just beginning to appear, preliminary experience is encouraging. New methods of screening can help to identify people who are at high risk for loss of independence. A brief period of care in a subacute unit may provide an opportunity to address the acute problems and to establish detailed plans for ongoing rehabilitation, good nutrition, and social support, thus averting the need to admit the patient to a hospital. Alternatively, brief subacute care may clarify that the patient is not a candidate to return home and should follow an appropriate pathway of long-term care. An admission to a subacute unit often provides excellent opportunities for health-related education of patients and families.

EVIDENCE OF EFFECTIVENESS OF SUBACUTE CARE

The regulations pertaining to subacute care reflect a fairly clear concept of what constitutes good comprehensive care for older patients. All the ingredients described above are ones that have emerged as essential components of good geriatrics care throughout the two or three decades of international experience in this field. It is not surprising, therefore, that subacute units have also been found to provide a useful environment for comprehensive assessment, especially for patients referred from community sites. The multidisciplinary staff, including medicine, nursing, social work, and the full range of rehabilitative specialties, coupled with a pace that is slower than that found in acute care hospitals, creates opportunities for conducting evaluations and formulating comprehensive care plans. One of the models of inpatient comprehensive geriatric assessment described in chapter 7 was studied in a subacute care unit (Applegate, Miller, & Graney, 1990).

Unfortunately, only two studies so far have compared the outcomes of subacute care with those of accredited rehabilitation facilities and skilled nursing facilities (Kane, Chen, Blewett & Sangl, 1996; Kramer et al., 1997). As chapter 9 describes in more detail, stroke patients achieved greater improvements following care in accredited rehabilitation units than in either of the other two settings. Stroke patients cared for in subacute units had outcomes similar to those cared for in skilled nursing facilities. The outcomes in patients with hip fractures did not consistently differ among any of the three types of facilities, except for more seriously ill patients, who fared best in the rehabilitation facilities (Kane et al., 1996). As described in chapter 9, preliminary data suggest similar rehabilitative outcomes in HMO subacute units and traditional FFS systems of care (Kramer, Kowalsky, Eilertsen, Hester, & Steiner, 1996).

Another report adds insight into some of the potential benefits of subacute care (vonSternberg et al., 1997). Outcome data were collected from 253 HMO enrollees with a variety of conditions who elected to receive post–acute care in subacute units in five nursing homes that contracted with the HMO. Investigators compared the outcomes of these patients with those of other HMO enrollees who elected to receive their post–acute care in community long-term institutions or rehabilitation units attached to hospitals. These units were not linked with the HMO's geriatric team through clinical participation or negotiated contract. The subacute patients received care as described above from an interdisciplinary team led by a board-certified geriatrician and a GNP. A rough comparison showed that in the subacute units, patients had an average length of stay of 14.3 days, while in the control facilities, the average was 20.5 days. Per diem costs were $185 for the subacute units and $280 to $300 for the control facilities.

Rehospitalization rates were the same, except that rehospitalization for infections was less frequent in the subacute facilities. Patients and providers in the subacute units reported high levels of satisfaction with their care.

SUMMARY

Subacute units constitute one of the fastest growing systems of care for older persons, offering care following hospitalization and also when direct admission from the community. None of the studies reported to date has used a randomized design, so drawing conclusions is difficult. Much more information is needed before the relative advantages and costs of rehabilitation facilities, skilled nursing facilities, and subacute units can be evaluated.

REFERENCES

Accreditation protocol for subacute programs. (1996). Oakbrook Terrace, IL: Joint Commission for the Accreditation of Health Care Organizations.

Applegate, W., Miller, S., Graney, M., Elan, J. T., Burns, R., & Adkins, D. E. (1990). A randomized controlled trial of geriatric assessment in a geriatric rehabilitation hospital. *New England Journal of Medicine, 322,* 1572–1578.

Kane, R. L., Chen, Q., Blewett, L. A., & Sangl, J. (1996). Do rehabilitative nursing homes improve the outcomes of care? *Journal of the American Geriatrics Society, 44,* 545–554.

Kramer, A. M., Kowalsky, J., Eilertsen, T. B., Hester, E. J., & Steiner, J. F. (1996, November). *Outcomes for stroke and hip fracture patients in HMO and fee-for-service systems.* Paper presented at Beyond the Waters Edge: Charting the Course of Managed Care for People With Disabilities, St. Michaels, MD.

Kramer, A., Steiner, J., Schlenker, R., Eilertsen, T., Hrincevich, C., Tropea, D., Ahmad, L., & Eckoff, D. (1997). Outcomes and costs after hip fracture and stroke. *Journal of the American Medical Association, 277,* 396–404.

Morrisey, M. A., Sloan, F. A., Valvona, J. (1988). Medicare prospective payment and posthospital transfers to subacute care. *Medical Care, 26,* 685–698.

Ouslander, J., Osterweil, D., & Morley, J. (1997). *Medical care in the nursing home* (2nd ed.). New York: McGraw-Hill.

von Sternberg, T., Hepburn, K., Cibuzar, P., Convery, L., Dokken, B., Haefemeyer, J., Rettke, S., Ripley, J., Rosenau, V., Rothe, P., Schurle, D., & WonSavage, R. (1997). Post-hospital subacute care: An example of a managed care model. *Journal of the American Geriatrics Society, 45,* 87–91.

9

Rehabilitation

Andrew M. Kramer

BACKGROUND

T. Franklin Williams, former director of the National Institute on Aging, described rehabilitation as "an approach, a philosophy, and a point of view as much as it is a set of techniques" (1984, p. 13). As in all of geriatrics, the approach and philosophy of rehabilitation are critical to achieving the goals of maximizing function and quality of life.

We generally use the term *rehabilitation* to refer to treatment following an acute event (e.g., stroke or hip fracture) aimed at restoring as much previous function as possible. The focus can be physical functioning, speech and language, and/or activities enabling an individual to return to the community. Following such an acute event, there is a window of opportunity, typically lasting between 3 and 6 months, within which rehabilitation is most beneficial (Duncan, Goldstein, Matchar, Divine, & Feussner, 1992; Magaziner, Simonsick, Kashner, Hebel, & Kenzora, 1990). Community-dwelling individuals usually return to the community within 90 days after a stroke or hip fracture; otherwise, they are likely to remain in a nursing home (Kramer, Steiner, Schlenker, Eilertsen, Hrincevich, Tropea, Ahmad, & Eckhoff, 1997).

Rehabilitation also plays a major role in treating chronic diseases among older persons. Such treatment may restore function lost from deconditioning caused by long-standing illness, such as cardiac or pulmonary disease. In geriatrics, however, we must broaden our view of rehabilitation to include services aimed at maintaining functional ability and avoiding the functional decline that could result from chronic disease.

The two most frequent events for which older people receive rehabilitation are stroke, with an incidence in the United States of approximately 550,000 per year, and hip fracture, with an incidence of about 250,000 per year (Gresham et al., 1995; Magaziner et al., 1990). Other fractures, arthropathies, and amputations are the next most common conditions, followed by neurologic diseases and other medical or surgical conditions such as cardiac, pulmonary, or neoplastic diseases. Physical disability is also caused by a wide range of other chronic illnesses (Kramer, Eilertsen, Hrincevich, & Schlenker, 1994).

The formulation of plans for rehabilitation must consider comorbid illnesses. Depression and cognitive impairment frequently accompany physical impairments from a stroke or hip fracture (Kramer, Steiner, Schlenker, et al., 1997; Mossey, Knott, & Craik, 1990). Identifying and treating depression leads to improved outcome, but depression frequently goes untreated (Anderson, Verstergaard, & Lauritzen, 1994; Gresham, et al., 1995). Similarly, hip fracture patients frequently have comorbid conditions that impair mobility (e.g., amputation) or interfere with the conditioning required for rehabilitation (e.g., pulmonary disease). Caregiving and social support can also be critical to rehabilitation outcomes (Cummings et al., 1988). Thus, geriatric rehabilitation requires a wide range of intensities and durations of therapy, as well as many supportive services.

Paradoxically, persons with the best function, fewest comorbidities, and greatest potential are most likely to receive the more comprehensive and intensive rehabilitation care (Kane, Chen, Blewett, & Sangl, 1996; Kramer, Steiner, Schlenker, et al., 1997). Rehabilitation care should not be forced on individuals who will not benefit, but we must guard against providing too little care to complex cases. Very small differences in functional improvement may determine whether a patient returns to a community residence or resides permanently in a nursing home.

REHABILITATION SETTINGS

Acute Hospital

After acute hospitals implemented the prospective payment system (PPS) and capitated managed care began, shorter lengths of stay substantially reduced the amount of rehabilitation that acute hospitals provided (Fitzgerald, Moore, & Dittus, 1988). There has been growing recognition, however, that the sooner elderly persons are mobilized and begin rehabilitation, the less conditioning they will lose and the fewer complications they will suffer (Gresham et al., 1995). Thus, rehabilitation services now begin earlier, but their duration in the acute hospital stay is shorter than in pre-PPS days.

Inpatient Rehabilitation Hospitals and Units

Medicare exempts certified rehabilitation hospitals and hospital units from the PPS and provides them instead with cost-based reimbursement for acute, physician-directed, interdisciplinary rehabilitation. To be eligible for this coverage, patients must have the potential for significant improvement and the capacity for at least 3 hours a day of physical, occupational, and/or speech therapy. Furthermore, at least 75% of the patients admitted to rehabilitation hospitals or units require services for 1 of 10 specified rehabilitation diagnoses (i.e., stroke, spinal cord injury, congenital deformities, amputations, multiple trauma, hip fracture, brain injury, polyarthritis, neurologic disorders, or burns).

Skilled Nursing Facilities (SNFs)

Recent estimates suggest that more than 70% of the 1.1 million Medicare-covered admissions to SNFs receive rehabilitation services (Kramer et al., 1994). Under fee-for-service Medicare, admission to the SNF requires a 3-day hospitalization within the previous 30 days. Therapy services must have a physician's order and be justified by improvement. Although Medicare covers up to 100 days of SNF care, it requires a large copayment after the 20th day. The amount and quality of both physician and rehabilitation services vary substantially among SNFs (Kramer, Schlenker, Eilertsen, & Hrincevich, 1997).

Home Health Agencies

Home health agencies provide rehabilitation services to homebound people who are making progress in recovering function. Home rehabilitation is covered by Medicare following either an acute hospital stay or an institutional rehabilitation episode (Lee, Huber, & Stason, 1996).

Comprehensive Outpatient Rehabilitation Facilities (CORF) and Outpatient Rehabilitation

A CORF is an outpatient facility that provides comprehensive diagnostic, therapeutic, and restorative services under physician direction; an outpatient rehabilitation center is a facility that provides any type of rehabilitation service. CORFs treated less than 1% of Medicare-covered stroke patients in 1991; hospital outpatient departments and independent ambulatory providers treated another 11% (Lee et al., 1996). As with rehabilitation hospitals and units, SNFs, and home health agencies, improvement must be documented; maintenance therapy is not reimbursed by Medicare.

SYSTEMS OF GERIATRIC REHABILITATION

Acute Hospital Rehabilitation Programs

The simplest intervention aimed at enhancing geriatric rehabilitation is the addition of professional expertise. A program tested in Britain involved moving elderly women with hip fractures to a rehabilitation ward where consultant geriatricians oversaw their care (Kennie, Reid, Richardson, Kiamari, & Kelt, 1988). In addition to the usual physical therapy, occupational therapy, orthopedic care, and medical attention, a consulting geriatrician made rounds and attended team meetings. A study showed patients who received such care had shorter rehabilitation times, were more likely at discharge to be independent in the activities of daily living, and were less likely to be discharged to long-term care institutions than recipients of standard rehabilitation. These beneficial effects were seen across a range of ages and mental states.

A similar hip fracture program in the United States involving an interdisciplinary team with a consulting internist/geriatrician demonstrated fewer postoperative complications and more improvement in ambulatory ability at hospital discharge (Zuckerman, Sakales, Fabian, & Frankel, 1992). This program focused on older hip fracture patients on a special hospital unit with dedicated staff, although it also provided a case manager for discharge planning and periodic contact with patients for 3 to 6 months.

Over the past two decades, researchers have extensively studied hospital-based stroke rehabilitation programs in the hospital, but the study designs have not always been rigorous, and the interventions have varied. A meta-analysis of 36 trials concluded that the average patient on a special stroke unit achieved better function than 66% of those on standard medical or neurologic units. The differences were greatest in randomized studies (Ottenbacher & Jannell, 1993).

Subacute Rehabilitation

A rapidly emerging alternative to hospital rehabilitation in the United States is subacute rehabilitation in SNFs (Kane et al., 1996; Manard et al., 1995). Such rehabilitation occurs in specialized units that provide services that are more comprehensive than those provided in the typical SNF. While these facilities have substantially fewer rehabilitation staff than rehabilitation hospitals and units, they have more staff than traditional nursing homes. Some subacute rehabilitation units receive higher reimbursement than traditional SNFs; some also have arrangements with physicians to provide more oversight. Typically, such programs make use of case management and clinical pathways.

Because of the recent emergence of subacute rehabilitation programs, we have relatively little evidence about their effectiveness and cost in comparison to traditional rehabilitation options. However, two national cohort studies compared outcomes achieved by subacute rehabilitation programs, traditional SNFs, and inpatient rehabilitation hospitals. One study of a national sample of 92 units or facilities from 17 states focused on patients with hip fractures or strokes (Kramer, Steiner, Schlenker, et al., 1997). After adjusting for risk factors, the rates of community residence and functional recovery at 6 months were the same for hip fracture patients, regardless of the type of rehabilitation program. However, stroke patients admitted to rehabilitation hospitals recovered the most function, and those admitted to subacute rehabilitation units or inpatient rehabilitation hospitals were more likely to be residing in the community at 6 months than those admitted to traditional nursing homes.

The second study included about 200 stroke patients and 370 hip fracture patients from three metropolitan areas. That study examined improvement in function 6 weeks, 6 months, and 12 months after hospital discharge (Kane at al., 1996). As in the first study, stroke patients admitted to inpatient rehabilitation hospitals had better functional outcomes than those admitted to either subacute or traditional nursing homes. Healthier hip fracture patients did not do quite as well in subacute units compared with rehabilitation facilities, but sample sizes were small in these subgroup analyses. A single site study of stroke patients also found greater functional improvement in an inpatient rehabilitation program than a subacute care program (Keith, Wilson, & Gutierrez, 1995).

In combination, these studies suggest that subacute rehabilitation may be as effective as rehabilitation hospital care for some conditions, such as hip fracture, but not as effective in terms of functional recovery in providing the complex interdisciplinary care required for stroke patients. Two studies found that subacute rehabilitation cost half as much per admission as hospital rehabilitation. Nevertheless, caution should accompany any use of subacute settings for complex rehabilitation.

Without any defined standards for subacute rehabilitation programs, the care that is provided in these settings varies substantially. Those programs that replicate much of the comprehensive rehabilitation that is available in the inpatient rehabilitation hospitals seem likely to be most successful in replicating the hospitals' functional outcomes. Some of the key services available in hospital settings—in addition to physical, occupational, and speech therapy—are recreational therapy, psychological services, and involvement of rehabilitation medicine physicians.

Some HMOs own or lease rehabilitative SNFs, which they staff at levels higher than even typical subacute SNFs (Kramer, Fox, & Morgenstern, 1992). In one such facility, the medical director and another full-time physician headed a team that admitted patients 7 days a week and followed them throughout their stay, visiting them several times a week (Kramer, Steiner, & Kowalsky, 1994). As discussed in Chapter 8, other HMOs contract with specific facilities and then bring in services to enhance subacute rehabilitative care (Kramer, Steiner, & Kowalsky, 1994; Von Sternberg et al., 1997). A national study is now comparing the outcomes achieved in six HMOs that use these comprehensive subacute units with those achieved in five vertically integrated care systems operating mostly under the fee-for-service Medicare program. Preliminary evidence suggests similar geriatric rehabilitation outcomes in both systems (Kramer, Kowalsky, Eilertsen, Hester, & Steiner, 1996).

Outpatient and Home Rehabilitation

Several studies have examined outpatient and home rehabilitation for stroke patients in the United Kingdom and New Zealand. Outpatient rehabilitation has not been shown to be more effective than usual care (Tucker, Davison, & Ogle, 1984), nor has it compared favorably with home rehabilitation (Young & Forster, 1992). There is also little evidence to suggest that traditional home rehabilitation improves functional recovery within the first 6 months (Wade, Langton-Hewer, Skilbeck, Bainton, & Burns-Cox, 1985). Intensive outpatient rehabilitation has been shown to be effective after stroke, but benefits decline after therapy stops (Wade, Collen, Robb, & Warlow, 1992). Thus, the evidence for the benefits of home and outpatient rehabilitation programs is weak.

Some HMOs have used intensive in-home rehabilitation. In one such program, Wellmark Healthcare treated over 500 patients in the Boston area (Portnow et al., 1991). They provided the full array of nursing, medical, and other rehabilitation services available in rehabilitation hospitals, requiring multiple home visits each day—in contrast to traditional home care with daily home visits and no home visits by physicians. While not rigorously evaluated, evidence collected by the agency suggests that it treats complex patients in the home with positive results.

Multiple Levels of Care

Some large, mature systems offer multiple levels of rehabilitation care. Such centers may provide rehabilitation care in a rehabilitation unit, a hospital-based SNF unit, an affiliated community-based SNF (under contract), a hospital-based home health agency, and an outpatient department. Patients make transitions among the settings as their needs change, and specialized staff such as rehabilitation medicine physicians or geriatricians consult across the various settings.

OUTLOOK

During the last decade, rehabilitation care has begun to shift out of the acute care hospital; by all signs, this will continue. While this movement, initiated largely to contain costs, is not necessarily a problem, we must be careful to maintain quality. Evidence suggests that for some conditions requiring complex interdisciplinary rehabilitation (e.g., stroke), outcomes that occur in the hospital setting may not transfer easily to other settings. In such cases, quality can probably be maintained only when sufficient expertise and funding are shifted from acute care to the alternative sites. Clinicians must advocate to ensure that these evolving options provide effective care.

One way to do this is to focus on the elements of care (e.g., care pathways, availability of services, service intensity, and service duration), rather than on the settings in which care is provided. We need to customize care to meet patients' needs, rather than compromising to meet the requirements and coverage policies of different settings. Therapy designed to avoid functional loss will require that low-intensity services be available over long intervals. This may also be necessary for frail older people who cannot tolerate multiple hours of therapy services each day, but who might regain some function or speech over an extended course of treatment.

Postacute care often lacks physicians' presence, despite evidence of beneficial effects. The evolution toward multiple transfers between settings during rehabilitation makes the presence of primary care physicians even more critical. While it may seem cost-effective to change settings when services that an individual requires can be met in a lower level of care, transitions from one setting to the next can create problems. For older persons and their families, transferring through multiple settings can be stressful and disorienting. Redundant evaluations and information transfers can compromise continuity of care. By actively managing the process, the primary care physician can minimize these problems.

As we move toward shorter stays and multiple transitions, the most insidious problem is the tendency to focus on individual segments of care rather than on the entire episode of rehabilitation. In this respect, capitated systems have a potential advantage over fee-for-service providers in that they are responsible for the whole continuum of rehabilitative services, whereas individual fee-for-service providers are more likely to focus more narrowly. Comprehensive rehabilitation ends only when the patient has reached a point of maximal recovery, perhaps 3 to 6 months after initiation; efforts to maintain function may last even longer. Future improvements in rehabilitative systems will depend on all providers assuming responsibility for the final outcome. Clinical pathways, outcome measures, and payments must be focused increasingly on the complete episode of care.

REFERENCES

Anderson, G., Vestergaard, K., & Lauritzen, L. (1994). Effective treatment of post-stroke depression with the selective serotonin reuptake inhibitor citalopram. *Stroke, 25,* 1099–1109.

Cummings, S. R., Phillips, S. L., Wheat, M. E., Black, D., Goosby, E., Wlodarczyk, D., Trafton, P., Jergesen, H., Winograd, C. H., & Hulley, S. B. (1988). Recovery of function after hip fracture: The role of social supports. *Journal of the American Geriatrics Society, 36,* 801–806.

Duncan, P. W., Goldstein, L. B., Matchar, D., Divine, G. W., & Feussner, J. (1992). Measurement of motor recovery after stroke: Outcome assessment and sample size requirements. *Stroke, 23,* 1084–1089.

Fitzgerald, J. F., Moore, P. S., & Dittus, R. S. (1988). The care of elderly patients with hip fracture: Changes since implementation of the prospective payment system. *New England Journal of Medicine, 319,* 1392–1397.

Gresham, G. E., Duncan, P. W., Stason, W. B., Adams, H. P., Adelman, A. M., Alexander, D. N., Bishop, D. S., Diller, L., Donaldson, N. E., Granger, C. V., Holland, A. L., Kelly-Hayes, M., McDowell, F. H., Myers, L., Phipps, M. A., Roth, E. J., Siebens, H. C., Tarvin, G. A., & Trombly, C. A. (1995). *Post-stroke rehabilitation* (Clinical Practice Guideline No. 16. AHCPR Publication No. 95-0662). Rockville, MD: U.S. Department of Health and Human Services, Public Health Service, Agency for Health Care Policy and Research.

Kane, R. L., Chen, Q., Blewett, L. A., & Sangl, J. (1996). Do nursing homes improve the outcomes of care? *Journal of the American Geriatrics Society, 44,* 545–554.

Keith, R. A., Wilson, D. B., & Gutierrez, P. (1995). Acute and subacute rehabilitation for stroke: A comparison. *Archives of Physical Medical Rehabilitation, 76,* 495–500.

Kennie, D. C., Reid, J., Richardson, I. R., Kiamari, A. A., & Kelt, C. (1988). Effectiveness of geriatric rehabilitative care of the proximal femur in elderly women: A randomized clinical trial. *British Medical Journal, 297,* 1083–1086.

Kramer, A. M., Eilertsen, T. B., Hrincevich, C. A., & Schlenker, R. E. (1994). *Study of the cost-effectiveness of subacute care alternatives and services: Rehabilitation of Medicare patients in rehabilitation hospitals and skilled nursing facilities.* Denver: Center for Health Services Research.

Kramer, A. M., Fox, P. D., & Morgenstern, N. (1992). Geriatric care approaches in health maintenance organizations. *Journal of the American Geriatric Society, 40,* 1055–1067.

Kramer, A. M., Kowalsky, J., Eilertsen, T. B., Hester, E. J., & Steiner, J. F. (1996, November). *Outcomes for stroke and hip fracture patients in HMO and fee-for-service systems.* Paper presented at Beyond the Waters Edge: Charting the Course of Managed Care for People With Disabilities, St. Michaels, MD.

Kramer, A. M., Schlenker, R. E., Eilertsen, T. B., & Hrincevich, C. A. (1997). Stroke rehabilitation in nursing homes. *Topics in Stroke Rehabilitation, 4,* 53–63.

Kramer, A. M., Steiner, J. F., & Kowalsky, J. (1994). Rehab for the elderly: An RWJ-funded project explores how six HMOs provide subacute and rehab care for the elderly. *HMO Magazine: Directions in Managed Care, 35,* 15–19.

Kramer, A. M., Steiner, J. F., Schlenker, R. E., Eilertsen, T. B., Hrincevich, C. A.,

Tropea, D. A., Ahmad, L. A., & Eckhoff, D. G. (1997). Outcomes and costs after hip fracture and stroke: A comparison of rehabilitation settings. *Journal of the American Medical Association, 277*, 396–404.

Lee, A. J., Huber, J. H., & Stason, W. B. (1996). Poststroke rehabilitation in older Americans: The Medicare experience. *Medical Care, 34*, 811–825.

Magaziner, J., Simonsick, E. M., Kashner, T. M., Hebel, J. R., & Kenzora, J. E. (1990). Predictors of functional recovery one year following discharge for hip fracture: A prospective study. *Journal of Gerontology, 45*, 101–107.

Manard, B., Bieg, K., Cameron, R., Junior, N., Kaplan, S., Keiller, A., & Perrone, C. (1995). *Subacute care: Policy synthesis and market area analysis.* Lewin-VHI. Washington D.C.

Mossey, J. M., Knott, K., & Craik, R. (1990). The effects of persistent depressive symptoms on hip fracture recovery. *Journal of Gerontology, 45*, 163–168.

Ottenbacher, K. J., & Jannell, S. (1993). The results of clinical trials in stroke rehabilitation research. *Archives of Neurology, 50*, 37–44.

Portnow, J., Kline, T., Daly, M., Peltier, S. M., Chin, C., & Miller, J. R. (1991). Multidisciplinary home rehabilitation: A practical model. *Clinics in Geriatric Medicine, 7*, 695–706.

Tucker, M. A., Davison, J. G., & Ogle, S. J. (1984). Day hospital rehabilitation—effectiveness and cost in the elderly: A randomized controlled trial. *British Medical Journal, 289*, 1209–1212.

Von Sternberg, T., Hepburn, K., Cibuzar, P., Convery, L., Dokken, B., Haefemeyer, J., Rettke, S., Ripley, J., Vosenau, V., Rother, P., Schurle, D., & Won-Savage, R. (1997). Post-hospital subacute care: An example of a managed care model. *Journal of the American Geriatrics Society, 45*, 87–91.

Wade, D. T., Collen, F. M., Robb, G. F., & Warlow C. P. (1992). Physiotherapy intervention late after stroke and mobility. *British Medical Journal, 304*, 609–613.

Wade, D. T., Langton-Hewer, R., Skilbeck, C. E., Bainton, D., & Burns-Cox, C. (1985). Controlled trial of a home-care service for acute stroke patients. *Lancet, 9*, 323–326.

Williams, T. F. (1984). *Rehabilitation in aging.* New York: Raven Press.

Young, J. B., & Forster, A. (1992). The Bradford community stroke trial: Results at six months. *British Medical Journal, 304*, 1085–1089.

Zuckerman, J. D. , Sakales, S. R. , Fabian, D. R. , & Frankel, V. H. (1992). Hip fractures in geriatric patients: Results of an interdisciplinary hospital care program. *Clinical Orthopedics and Related Research, 274*, 213–225.

10

Care of Older People Who Are Dying

Robert M. McCann

BACKGROUND

Providing care for dying persons and their families may be one of the greatest challenges that physicians and health care providers face. The delivery of excellent palliative care demands in-depth knowledge of the patient's social supports, spiritual beliefs, and finances, in addition to his or her medical problems. Health systems that support the multidisciplinary requirements of palliative care are essential to the delivery of quality care.

The Current State of End-of-Life Care

While medical care often slows the course of dying, modern medicine has devoted little attention to how patients live while they are dying. Most older persons die in hospitals and nursing homes and experience considerable discomfort, typically being exposed to considerable amounts of invasive, life-sustaining therapies (Lynn et al., 1997; McCue, 1995). The increased use of technology and the "war" mentality toward various diseases have stimulated an increased tendency to intervene, even when a favorable outcome is only remotely possible. An implicit value to "doing something" has fueled an increasing use of high-technology resources for dying persons. End-of-life care utilizes an estimated 10% of our health care resources (Scitovsky, 1994). With overwhelming evidence of ineffective care at the end of life, one must question whether these resources are being well spent.

A recent large study of severely ill, hospitalized patients showed that 50% of patients who died experienced moderate to severe pain for the last 3 days of their lives (SUPPORT Principal Investigators, 1995). This occurred despite the fact that the tools and the knowledge for adequate treatment of pain have been available for many years. When applied appropriately, current treatment modalities are almost uniformly success-ful in relieving the majority of pain in terminally ill patients. Other stud-ies also have demonstrated ineffective pain control and symptom pallia-tion in dying persons. (Cleeland et al., 1994; Foley, 1995; "Good Care," 1996; Lynn, Teno et al., 1997; Max, 1990). The SUPPORT study demon-strated that many dying patients also received invasive medical interven-tions that were inconsistent with their wishes as indicated by advance directives. It also showed that a nurse-mediated attempt to improve com-munications between physicians and dying patients was ineffective. While hospital systems have gained increasing expertise in highly tech-nological interventions for acute care, they have had much less incentive to develop systems that enhance the delivery of excellent palliative care.

Hospice Care

Hospice may be the best example of a system of care that has substantially improved the life of dying persons. The hospice movement began in 1967 at St. Christopher Hospice in London. Medicare began covering hospice benefits for its beneficiaries in 1982. The hospice philosophy introduced patient-centered, multidisciplinary care to dying patients, while focusing attention on how to improve dying persons' lives during their final days. Hospice philosophy embodies several concepts (Schonwetter, 1996):

1. Death is a natural part of the life cycle. When death is inevitable, hospice staff will neither seek to hasten nor postpone it.
2. Pain relief and symptom control are the primary clinical goals.
3. Psychological and spiritual pain are as significant as physical pain, and addressing all three requires the skills of an interdisciplinary team.
4. The unit of care comprises patients, their families, and loved ones.
5. Bereavement care is critical to supporting surviving family members and friends.
6. Care is provided regardless of ability to pay.

The hospice interdisciplinary team includes the attending physician, hospice physician, nurse, social worker, spiritual counselor, aides, volun-teers, and, when needed, physical, occupational and speech therapists, and psychiatrists.

Despite improved outcomes demonstrated by hospice care, patients still tend to enter these programs very near the end of their lives, thus missing some of the potential benefits of this type of care. Hospice care in the United States has tended to center on home care with short periods of institutional respite in hospitals or nursing homes (Schonwetter, 1996). Nursing homes and community care homes increasingly utilize the services of hospices to enhance their care of dying persons, enabling them to provide more one-on-one care using hospice nurses and aides, to seek consultation on pain control and other palliative measures from an expert team, to educate staff, and to provide bereavement counseling to families after the death. Financial benefits include assistance with the cost of medications and medical equipment directly related to the terminal disease suffered by the patient. For a patient to be eligible for hospice care, a physician must deem the patient to have a life expectancy of less than 6 months.

The National Hospice Organization has recently published a manual for determining prognosis in noncancer diseases (Standards and Accreditation Committee, 1996). Documents like this help clinicians estimate the prognosis for illnesses not typically thought of as "terminal," such as Alzheimer's disease. The use of such tools hopefully will increase the number of persons being referred to and benefiting from hospice care.

Other advances in palliative care include palliative care units, centers for pain control, journals specifically focused on palliative care, and a variety of medical, social, and ethical professionals who specialize in palliative care.

ENHANCING QUALITY AT THE END OF LIFE

Advance Directives

The doctrine of informed consent enforces the right to bodily control and promotes informed refusal of therapies and interventions. A mentally competent person has the right to refuse any therapy. The physician should provide guidance, but the ultimate decision belongs to the patient. This emphasis on patient autonomy has evolved over the years from a system of paternalism. When the patient loses the capacity to decide, the right to refuse transfers to a surrogate decision maker.

Advance care directives allow patients to express the type of care that they would desire were they to lose their capacity to participate in their medical decisions. The specification of what patients value in life and the circumstances under which life might not be worth living can be very useful when deciding on treatments for patients who lose their decision-making capacity.

Lack of specificity in the advance directives themselves and the difficulty of predicting what one might want in the future often limit the usefulness of written directives in clinical practice. Completion rates of advance directives remain low (10% to 15%) (Johnston, Pfeifer, & McNutt, 1995; Silverman & Blanken, 1996), despite the enactment of the Patient Self-Determination Act of 1991, which requires institutions to provide information to patients regarding advance directives. Unfortunately, the multitude of documents in hospital admission packets often obscures the presence of this information. One study showed that providing advance directives to patients before planned admissions increased the completion rate from 4% to 40% (Cugliari, Miller, & Sobal, 1995).

Even when advance directives are completed, they are often not available to or followed by health care providers. In the SUPPORT study (1995), providers wrote do not resuscitate orders for only 52% of patients who preferred not to be resuscitated. Advance directive documents often are not accessible when patients move from ambulatory or nursing home care to hospitals.

To systematically increase the completion and effectiveness of advance directives:

- patients should receive, preferably in ambulatory care settings prior to sentinel events, meaningful and understandable information regarding informed consent for medical interventions at the end of life
- information systems should integrate advance directive documents across acute, chronic, and ambulatory care settings
- research and quality assurance interventions should consider enhancing patient-physician communication about end-of-life decisions.

Preventing Harm

The transition from life-prolonging care to palliative care is difficult for patients and for health care providers. Interventions such as cardiopulmonary resuscitation (CPR) have no place in the care of terminally ill patients. CPR is relatively ineffective in frail older persons having irreversible functional dependence. Two studies that examined the outcomes of patients living in nursing homes who received CPR followed by hospital admission showed that less than 4% survived to hospital discharge, often more debilitated than before experiencing cardiac arrest (Gordon & Cheung, 1993; Murphy, Murray, Robinson, & Campion, 1989). What was initially a therapy to prevent sudden death from acute myocardial infarction has become the default treatment for any death.

Other "routine" medical treatments, such as antibiotic therapy, are also often inappropriate in the care of dying patients. Since most terminally ill persons eventually succumb to infection, treatment of infections may only prolong a patient's suffering and must be carefully considered in the context of the patient's prognosis, goals, and values.

CONCLUSION

Improving the quality of care at the end of life demands a thoughtful, systematic series of interventions. These interventions must

- enhance physician-patient communication
- educate the public about palliative care and the sometimes unrealistic expectations of medical care to prevent all death and disease
- provide meaningful informed consent regarding medical treatment choices at the end of life
- educate professionals about the importance and the methods of providing excellent palliative care at the end of life
- ensure that finances and payment sources encourage and do not discourage excellent palliative care

Broad-reaching interventions such as these are more likely to take place in health systems that understand the importance of multidisciplinary care and are committed to providing excellent palliative care.

REFERENCES

Cleeland, C. S., Gonin, R., Hatfield, A. K, Edmonson, J. H., Blum, R., Stewart, J. A., & Pandya, K. J. (1994). Pain and its treatment in outpatients with metastatic cancer. *New England Journal of Medicine, 330,* 592–596.

Cugliari, A. M., Miller, T., & Sobal, J. (1995). Factors promoting completion of advance directives in the hospital. *Archives of Internal Medicine, 155,* 1893–1898.

Foley, K. M. (1995). Pain relief into practice: Rhetoric without reform. *Journal of Clinical Oncology, 13,* 2149–2151.

Good care of the dying patient. (1996). *Journal of the American Medical Association, 275,* 474–478.

Gordon, M., & Cheung, M. (1993). Poor outcome of on-site CPR in a multi-level geriatric facility: Three and a half years' experience at the Baycrest Centre for geriatric care. *Journal of the American Medical Association, 41,* 163–166.

Johnston, S. C., Pfeifer. M. P., & McNutt, R. (1995). The discussion about advance directives. *Archives of Internal Medicine, 155,* 1025–1030.

Lynn, J., Teno, J., Phillips, R. S., Wu, A. W., Desbiens, N., Kreling, B., & Connors, A. F. (1997). Perceptions by family members of the dying experience of older and seriously ill patients. *Annals of Internal Medicine, 126,* 97–106.

Max, M. (1990). Improving outcomes of analgesia treatment: Is education enough? *Annals of Internal Medicine, 113,* 885–889.

McCue, J. (1995). The naturalness of dying. *Journal of the American Medical Association, 273,* 1039–1042.

Murphy, D., Murray, A., Robinson, B., & Campion, E. (1989). Outcomes of cardiopulmonary resuscitation in the elderly. *Annals of Internal Medicine, 111,* 199–205.

Schonwetter, R. (1996). Care of the dying geriatric patient. In *Care of the Terminally Ill Patient: Clinics in Geriatric Medicine, 12,* 253–265.

Scitovsky, A. A. (1994). The high cost of dying revisited. *Milbank Quarterly, 72,* 561–592.

Silverman, H. J., & Blanken, P. N. (1996). Advanced directives: Are they fulfilling their purpose? *Current Opinions in Critical Care, 2,* 337–343.

Standards and Accreditation Committee. (1996). *Medical guidelines for determining prognosis in selected non-cancer diseases* (2nd ed.). Arlington, VA: Medical Guidelines Task Force of the National Hospice Organization.

SUPPORT Principal Investigators. (1995). A controlled trial to improve care for seriously ill hospitalized patients: The study to understand prognoses and preferences for outcomes and risks of treatments (SUPPORT). *Journal of the American Medical Association, 274,* 1591–1598.

IV

When the Older Person Is Disabled

*T*he numbers are staggering. Currently in the United States, there are about 5 million elderly community dwellers who need long-term care and approximately 2 million nursing home residents. By 2030, these figures will rise to about 12 million noninstitutionalized and 4 million institutionalized older adults requiring long-term care. The challenges of long-term care are mainly posed by the most rapidly growing population segment: Half of persons age 85 and over require assistance with their daily activities.

Many of the challenges in acute and chronic care are magnified in long-term care. Medically, older adults requiring long-term care are more frail, usually having accumulated several chronic conditions. Previously episodic health events and periodic medical contacts become almost daily occurrences. Psychosocially, long-term care dramatically threatens the autonomy of those affected. The greater the disability and need for daily assistance, the more long-term care intrudes upon the lives of those affected; the nursing home represents the most extreme example of this, where older adults must give up their own home and move into a place specifically designed for their care. Financially, the spiraling costs of long-term care services present huge individual and societal burdens.

Most older adults requiring long-term care reside in the community. The first two chapters of this section focus on defining the complex taxonomy of community-based long-term care and its effects on patient outcomes and cost. The next chapter deals with systems of care for those affected by Alzheimer's disease, a condition that poses huge challenges by virtue of its high prevalence, chronicity, and propensity to cause progressive disability. Finally, the state-of-the-art and future of nursing home care are addressed.

11

Overview of Community-Based Long-Term Care

Amasa B. Ford

INTRODUCTION

Dramatic increases in human longevity point to long-term care as one of the great challenges of the 21st century. Somewhat surprisingly, as we examine the problem, we find that, even as in colonial days, family and friends still provide the bulk of such care, in the home. We can no longer equate long-term care with what happens in nursing homes, and we now ask whether an institution is the most appropriate place to die.

Some fundamental questions arise: What is long-term care? Which persons need such care? Where do they seek it? How do the processes of long-term care operate? And, finally, how can we improve the final outcome? Although seemingly chaotic, the "system" of long-term care does have a structure and operates through several familiar processes, even though disagreement surrounds the method of evaluating the outcome of these processes (see chapter 5).

HOW DO WE DEFINE THE NEED FOR LONG-TERM CARE?

Long-term care, broadly speaking, is a response to the presence of chronic conditions or diseases and the disabilities they cause. For the purposes of this chapter, a more focused definition is, simply, services for those who can no longer function independently. We usually define the measurement of functional status in terms of reported ability to perform basic activities of daily living (ADLs) and instrumental activities (IADLs), such as meal preparation (Wiener, Hanley, Clark, & VanNostrand, 1990).

WHO NEEDS LONG-TERM CARE?

A distinction between chronic conditions and functional limitations helps to clarify the picture. Of 26 million noninstitutionalized persons age 65 years and older who were living in the United States in 1987, 23 million (82%) reported that they had at least one chronic condition, and 16 million (62%) reported two or more such conditions (Hoffman, Rice, & Sung, 1996). In terms of functional limitation, however, Medicare classified only 12.8% as limited in the performance of activities of daily living (Laschober & Olin, 1996).

We can apply these percentages to an estimated 1996 population of 34 million older persons and arrange them on a continuum of incremental need for care: 9.6 million (28%) were well, 18.6 million (55%) resided in the community with chronic conditions but without functional limitations, 4.1 million (12%) resided in the community with chronic conditions and limitations, and 1.7 million (5%) resided in institutions and suffered from both chronic conditions and functional limitations. Thus, less than 30% of the older persons who were sick and disabled received institutional care.

WHERE DO OLDER PERSONS SEEK CARE?

To answer this question, we must examine the entire pattern of health behavior of the older population. Figure 11.1 summarizes data from many sources and includes some estimates and approximations. It depicts a dynamic system animated by constant flows of individuals through offices, clinics, hospitals and nursing homes, and, often, back to the community. The institutions are shown in black; the arrows represent changes in status and location, and exit from the system is shown below as the true "bottom line." The preponderance of older persons live in the community, whereas at the end of life most die in institutions (82% either in hospitals or in nursing homes). In addition, 14% die at home under hospice care, and 4% die outside of institutions or hospice (the latter figure not shown in Figure 11.1). The dynamic character of the "system" is impressive. For example, it is not generally recognized that, every year, more than a half million elderly persons enter nursing homes from the community, enter nursing homes from hospitals, or die in nursing homes, while more than a quarter million die at home, with a majority of these enrolled in a hospice program.

Comparing these figures with 1975 and 1985 data, significant trends appear (Ford, 1986, 1992). While the U.S. population increased 8.5 % over 15 years, the elderly population grew by 28%. More older persons died in

Older Persons and the Health Care System
(All figures in thousands)

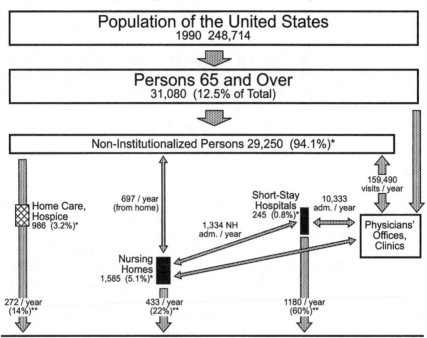

Population of the United States
1990 248,714

Persons 65 and Over
31,080 (12.5% of Total)

Non-Institutionalized Persons 29,250 (94.1%)*

Home Care, Hospice
986 (3.2%)*

697 / year
(from home)

1,334 NH
adm. / year

Nursing Homes
1,585 (5.1%)*

Short-Stay Hospitals
245 (0.8%)*

10,333
adm. / year

159,490
visits / year

Physicians' Offices, Clinics

272 / year
(14%)**

433 / year
(22%)**

1180 / year
(60%)**

All Deaths - - - 1,966 / Year

* - % of Older Persons
** - % of Deaths

FIGURE 11.1 Location and flow of older persons through the health care system in the United States, 1990. Some numbers are estimates or interpolations. Sources: Population: U.S. Bureau of the Census, 1990 Census of Population, 1993. Office visits: National Center for Health Statistics (NCHS), Vital and Health Statistics, Series 10, No. 181, 1991. Hospitals: NCHS, Vital and Health Statistics, Series 13, No. 112, 1992; NCHS, National Hospital Discharge Survey, personal communication. Nursing homes: NCHS, Vital and Health Statistics, Series 13 No. 102, 1989, and No. 103, 1990; NCHS, Advance Data No. 289, 1997. Home and hospice care: NCHS, Vital and Health Statistics, Series 13, No. 117, 1994, and No. 126, 1997; Advance Data No. 287, 1997. Deaths: Vital Statistics of the United States, 1989, Vol. 2, 1993; NCHS, Vital and Health Statistics, Series 13, No. 112, 1990.

hospitals and fewer died in nursing homes in 1990 than in 1975, but the proportion dying at home has remained almost constant. While the numbers of older persons in hospitals on a given day have changed very little, the nursing home population has increased by 41%—a trend that would be financially ruinous to maintain.

Strikingly, the community stands out as the source, the receiver, and the residence of most chronically ill older persons. On the other hand, institutions, particularly hospitals, which house so many of our resources, personnel, and technology, deliver a critical but limited part of long-term care on an increasingly transient basis.

HOW DO THE PROCESSES OF LONG-TERM CARE OPERATE?

Careers in long-term care can range from lifelong institutionalization to near-complete independence right to the end, but most people come to depend on some form of long-term care for months or years. By one estimated average, women age 65 years in 1991 could expect to live 18.6 more years, three quarters of that time independent of services. Men age 65, in contrast, could expect to live only 14.4 more years, but 83% of those years would be independent (Manton & Stallard, 1991). Of those who survive to age 85, 50% of the men and 70% of women can expect to spend some time in a nursing home (Murtaugh, Kemper, Spillman, & Carlson, 1997).

Hospitals and nursing homes provide some long-term care services, although even these apparently stable institutions are changing rapidly in response to market forces. Three quarters of long-term care for noninstitutionalized older persons, however, comes from spouses, other family members and occasionally from friends, supplemented by an array of supportive services that is developing belatedly in the United States. We shall briefly survey now the main types of long-term care.

COMMUNITY SERVICES

Community services provide the bulk of long-term care. Older persons who are well (28% of older persons) and those with identified chronic conditions but no functional limitations (55%) often do not view themselves as sick or disabled. Some take advantage of the health maintenance, diagnostic, screening, and primary prevention procedures (see chapters 1 and 2), but many who could benefit from well-established procedures do not receive them.

The older persons who live in the community and have both chronic conditions and functional limitations (12% of older persons) will most likely seek care from physicians or clinics, in the form of treatment, rehabilitation, and secondary prevention services (see chapters 3 and 9). Hospitals used to provide many of these services, such as establishing programs for newly identified diabetics or initiating poststroke rehabilitation; now, economic pressures dictate that patients seek help from nursing home, rehabilitation, ambulatory, or home care services. Again, the burden of furnishing such services falls mainly on the primary care physician, his or her historically new allies, the physician assistant and the nurse practitioner, and on the emerging teams who provide organized comprehensive care (chapter 16).

The care of the dying, another important component of long-term care, is at last receiving regard and moving out of the fast-paced hospital into the greater calm of the home, where most aged people believe it belongs. The hospice movement has grown remarkably in the past decade (Schonwetter, 1996). Chapter 10 presents the hospice concept and how it has evolved in concert with other supportive services, most of which are based in the community. These combined services explicitly aim to avoid institutionalization when possible. Hospice programs do well in achieving this goal, since only 7% of persons admitted to hospice programs die in a hospice institution or in a hospital (Haupt, 1997).

INSTITUTIONAL SERVICES

Conventional wisdom has long placed the nursing home as the primary provider of long-term care. As Figure 11.1 suggests, a substantial number of older persons circulate among homes, nursing homes, hospitals, and other institutions. As described in chapter 14, the nursing home of the future logically will evolve to be the hub of a network of community-based services (Burton, 1994; Ford, 1995). A much more active interchange between new-style nursing homes and the community has already begun to develop, with associated day care, respite care, and coordinated home care supplementing traditional care provided in the nursing home itself.

The need for less costly community-based alternatives to nursing home care has led in two different directions. One is the PACE program, an organized system of comprehensive support for sick and disabled older persons living in their own homes, paid for by Medicare and Medicaid (see chapter 16). The other is the unplanned proliferation of small "board and care homes," which are twice as numerous as nursing homes but accommodate less than a third the number of residents (Sirrocco, 1994). Board and care homes have emerged informally outside the "system," but they are now being licensed and regulated in several states and probably will evolve as a type of nursing home.

For such a community-based long-term care system to realize its full potential, many existing barriers must fall. Transfers between hospitals and nursing homes, in both directions, must become smoother and better planned. Older people living in the community also need wide-ranging transportation systems. Assisted living quarters and residential facilities designed for older and disabled persons now conjoin with nursing homes, forming retirement communities with shared central services. Up to this point, recipients of coordinated multilevel services have been mainly affluent persons, but lower-income persons need these services just as much.

Finally, hospitals are critical components of the long-term care network (see chapter 7). Although, in the past, hospitals have been oriented to acute care and, in fact, have managed acute events in the course of lengthy illnesses or disability, the average age of hospital patients has risen faster than would be indicated by the aging of the population. As infections and acute illnesses become more controllable, hospital functions diverge toward coping with clinical events that produce disability, such as hip fractures or strokes, or toward rehabilitative measures that may be considered part of long-term care, such as coronary bypass surgery or joint replacement.

These changes in the function of the modern hospital, however, have produced a highly technical environment that is in many ways unfriendly to the complex needs and slower adjustment of the elderly person. Growing consensus embraces the notion that older persons are better served if they leave the hospital as soon as possible or avoid hospitalization altogether. Chapter 7 describes programs that minimize the harm hospitalization frequently inflicts on older persons. In addition, the newly emerging hospital-affiliated rehabilitation units (see chapter 9), although initially stimulated by economic forces, may prove to provide a pace and environment in which older persons can begin to recuperate from a medical catastrophe. Here again, the interface between the institution and the community is changing. If all goes well, the agonizing choice between discharge to home (for which the patient and family often were not prepared) and discharge to a nursing home (implying permanent disability) will succumb to a friendlier, more flexible set of options, better adapted to the individual's specific needs.

IMPLICATIONS: HOW CAN WE IMPROVE THE OUTCOME?

First, an improved system must meet the needs of older people as well as those of institutions and providers. This goal implies a greater respect for individual choice and autonomy. Planning for services must weigh in location, transportation, housing, and other physical and emotional needs, in addition to simply striving to provide the most up-to-date and efficient medical care.

Second, a different, more egalitarian array of professional service providers will be needed. Primary care physicians have finally received recognition as the logical basis for a rational system, but we already risk placing too much responsibility on them. Primary physicians must be willing and enabled, in turn, to collaborate effectively with their necessary colleagues—nurses, social workers, and therapists—and, above all, with the people whom they serve. Volunteers, particularly those serving as family caregivers, must also be recognized as respected members of the team.

This overview has highlighted the fragmentary, incomplete, and sometimes incoherent nature of our present "system" and its many different roots. The present management crisis, although painfully antithetical to the essentially altruistic foundation of health care, may yet have a bright side. In redesigning the components of health care to be more cost-efficient, we may—through integration, coordination, and communication—be able to produce a true system that is simultaneously user-friendly, cost-effective, and medically sound.

REFERENCES

Burton, J. R. (1994). The evolution of nursing homes into comprehensive geriatrics centers: A perspective. *Journal of the American Geriatrics Society, 42,* 794–796.

Ford, A. B. (1986). The aged and their physicians. In E. Calkins, P. J. Davis, & A. B. Ford, A. B. (Eds.) *The practice of geriatrics* (p. 10). Philadelphia: Saunders.

Ford, A. B. (1992). The aged and their physicians. In E. Calkins, P. J. Davis, & A. B. Ford (Eds.), *The practice of geriatrics* (2nd ed., p. 6). Philadelphia: Saunders.

Ford, A. B. (1995). Long-term care: A new model. In P. R. Katz & M. D. Mezey (Eds.), *Quality care in geriatric settings: Focus on ethical issues.* New York: Springer, pp. 37–46.

Haupt, B. J. (1997). Characteristics of hospice care discharges: United States, 1993–94 (Advance Data No. 287). Hyattsville, MD: U.S. Department of Health and Human Services, National Center for Health Statistics.

Hoffman, C., Rice, D., & Sung, H. (1996). Persons with chronic conditions: Their prevalence and costs. *Journal of the American Medical Association, 276,* 1473–1479.

Laschober, M. A., & Olin, G. L. (1996). *Health and health care of the Medicare population: Data from the 1992 Current Beneficiary Survey.* Rockville, MD: Westat.

Manton, K. G., & Stallard, E. (1991). Cross-sectional estimates of active life expectancy for the U.S. elderly and oldest-old populations. *Journals of Gerontology: Social Sciences, 46,* S170–S182.

Murtaugh, C. M., Kemper, P., Spillman, B. C., & Carlson, B. L. (1997). The amount, distribution and timing of lifetime nursing home use. *Medical Care, 35,* 204–218.

Schonwetter, R. S. (1996). Care of the dying patient. In R. S. Schonwetter (Ed.), *Clinics in geriatric medicine* (Vol. 12, pp. 417–428). Philadelphia: Saunders.

Sirrocco, A. (1994). *Nursing homes and board and care homes: Data from the 1991 National Health Provider Inventory* (Advance Data No. 244). Hyattsville, MD: U.S. Department of Health and Human Services, National Center for Health Statistics.

Wiener, J. M., Hanley, R. J., Clark, R., & VanNostrand, J. F. (1990). Measuring the activities of daily living: Comparison across national surveys. *Journals of Gerontology: Social Sciences, 45,* S229–S237.

12

Outcomes and Costs of Home and Community-Based Long-Term Care: Implications for Research-Based Practice

William G. Weissert and Susan C. Hedrick

Very few health care interventions have been as well studied as community-based long-term care programs (CBLTC). A total of 36 well-designed studies have now been conducted of such programs as home care, adult day health care, and coordinated packages of services. In this chapter, we update our previous paper (Weissert & Hedrick, 1994), which in turn was based on a rigorous review of this literature (Weissert, Cready, & Pawelak, 1988, 1989), and draw lessons that can be gleaned from this large body of work.

The need for further dissemination of these results and their implications is evident: Of the 36 studies, only 3 were published in clinical journals and none in geriatrics journals. In his history of home care policy in the United States, Benjamin (1993) remarks on the curious persistence of claims that home care produces cost savings and the reliance on these claims to legitimize the programs, even when the "most consistent theme

* This chapter is based, with modification, on an article "Lessons learned from research on effects of community based long-term care," Weissert WG and Hedrick, SC, 1994 *Journal of the American Geriatrics Society, 42,* 348–353 with permission from the publisher.

in home care research" has been that such claims could not be supported. Increased exposure to this literature is important in informing the debates about the place of community-based long-term care in ongoing health care reforms.

The continued popularity of these programs in the absence of demonstrated cost-effectiveness provides a message that "it may be time to lay aside studies showing that home care is not cost-effective and get started on ways to make it become so" (Weissert, 1990 pp: 42–44). Here we do so by using the results of our own and others' syntheses of the prior research on this type of care to offer advice on how to make it cost-effective.

We updated our literature review using a rigorous procedure for study selection and review with explicit methodological criteria for validity and generalizability (Petersen & White, 1989). Studies reviewed evaluated a wide variety of programs, including in-home nursing or interdisciplinary team care (Bergner, et al., 1988; Hanchett & Torrens, 1967; Hughes, Cordray, & Spiker, 1984; Hughes et al., 1990, 1992; Katz, Ford, Downs, Adams, & Rusby, 1972; Melin, Hakansson, & Bygren, 1993; Papsidero, Katz, Kroger, & Akpom, 1979; Posman, Kogan, LeMat, & Dahlin, 1964; Selmanoff, Mitchell, Widlock, & Mossholder, 1979; Wade, Langton-Hewer, Skilbeck, Bainton, & Burns-Cox, 1985; Zimmer, Groth-Junker, & McCusker, 1985), homemaker or home aide care (Blenkner, Bloom, Nielsen, & Beggs, 1970; Nielsen, Blenkner, Bloom, Downs, & Beggs, 1972; Weissert, Wan, Livieratos, & Katz, 1980), adult day health care (Eagle et al., 1991; Hedrick et al., 1993; Weissert, Wan, Livieratos, & Pellegrino, 1980), hospice (Kane, Wales, Bernstein, Leibowitz, & Kaplan, 1984; Mor, Greer, & Kastenbaum, 1988), respite care (Lawton, Brody, & Saperstein, 1989), and programs that provide a coordinated package of these and other services (Berkeley Planning Associates, 1987; Birnbaum, Gaumer, Pratter, & Burke, 1984; Blenkner, Bloom, & Nielsen, 1971; Brown, Blackman, Learner, Witherspoon, & Saber, 1985; Commonwealth of Massachusetts, 1975; Gaumer et al., 1986; Kemper, 1988; Maurer, Ross, & Bigos, 1984; Oktay & Volland, 1986; O'Rourke, Raisz, & Segal, 1982; Pinkerton & Hill, 1984; Sainer, Brill, & Horwitz, 1984; Seidl, Applebaum, Austin, & Mahoney, 1983; Skellie, Favor, Tudor, & Strauss, 1982; Sklar & Weiss, 1983; Weissert, Lesnick, Musliner, & Foley, 1997; Zawadski, Shen, Yordi, & Hansen, 1984).Studies completed to date have not evaluated the cost-effectiveness of short-term "high technology" post–acute care provided in the home. In several cases, studies contained two distinct substudies of different populations, published separately and treated as different studies here, making a total of 38 studies reviewed.

We limited this review to studies using randomized controlled trials or quasi-experimental designs. (In the latter, results for a matched comparison group are compared to the treatment group.) These designs are critical, as they control for the fact that some patients will get better and others worse regardless of care, and they control for bad guesses about what care patients would have used had they not received CBLTC. A common weakness in studies with other designs is that they speculate that patients would have gone into nursing homes for long stays, calculate what they would have spent, then subtract CBLTC costs and claim savings. But randomized trials have proved that most patients would not go to nursing homes even if they did not receive CBLTC. Meta-analyses and reviews of this literature find that randomized controlled trials are associated with weaker effects of the intervention than nonrandomized trials (Hedrick, Koepsell, & Inui, 1989; Hughes et al., 1997; Weissert et al., 1988).

The studies reviewed employed a broad range of measures of patient and informal caregiver outcomes that include all of the major domains of quality of life seen as important in clinical trials (Grannemann, Grossman, & Dunstand, 1986). Outcomes measured include survival; physical and mental functioning; life satisfaction; social functioning; unmet needs; informal caregiver (e.g., spouse) support, function, and burden; satisfaction with care; utilization of health care; the costs of those services, including nursing homes, hospitals, and outpatient care; and out-of-pocket and caregiver time costs.

HEALTH OUTCOMES

The results of these studies have been remarkably robust and consistent, varying little in spite of variation in study dates, locations, populations, measures, frequency and duration of observations, data analytic methods, and services provided. We first summarize the results for the whole study groups, then discuss the results for subgroups of patients.

The studies show that in almost all cases, CBLTC does not increase survival and does not reverse or slow the rate of deterioration in functional status (see Table 12.1). Some studies observe a reduction in unmet needs; a few observed improved patient and caregiver life satisfaction. However, the higher life satisfaction levels tend to diminish and disappear over a few months despite continued use of CBLTC services.

The results are even more consistent among the studies that used the most rigorous research designs, largest samples, and most appropriate methods of analysis, including analysis of deleted cases. For example, only two of the studies that found a significant positive effect on survival were randomized controlled trials, and only one of those used multivariate analyses. An earlier meta-analysis of a subset of this literature did not find a significant survival effect but found that positive survival effects were associated with nonrandomized trials (Hedrick et al., 1989).

TABLE 12.1   Effects of Community-Based Long-Term Care

Outcome* or Utilization	Number of Studies	Results		
		Positive and Significant**	Negative and Significant**	Not Significant
Survival	30	7	1	22
ADL	34	3	4	27
IADL	15	3	3	9
Mobility	16	1	2	13
Restricted days	5	0	0	5
Mental functioning	29	3	0	26
Life satisfaction	24	5	1	18
Social activity	17	4	0	13
Social interaction	19	3	1	15
Unmet needs	35	21	0	14
Informal support	53	6	5	42
Caregiver satisfaction, stress, illness, etc.	18	4	1	13
Nursing home admission	16	5***	0***	11
Nursing home days	30	8***	1***	11
Hospital admission	13	2***	2***	9
Hospital days	23	7***	0***	16

* Multiple instruments were used to measure these outcomes across studies. If a study employed more than one measure of an outcome, each measure is counted separately here.
** Significance at $p \leq 0.05$.
*** "Positive" indicates treatment group had significantly fewer patients admitted/patient days than control group; "negative" indicates the reverse.
Sources: Bergner et al., 1988; Eagle, Guyatt, & Patterson, 1991; Hedrick et al., 1993; Hughes, et al., 1990; 19992; Lawton, Brady, & Saperstein, 1991; Melin, Hakansson, & Byrgren, 1993; Weissert, Cready, & Pawelak, 1988; Weissert, Lesnick, Musliner, & Foley, in press.

EFFECTS ON HEALTH CARE UTILIZATION AND COST

Only a few studies observed a decrease in the use of nursing homes and hospitals. The decreases were too small to outweigh the costs of the additional CBLTC services, resulting in an overall rise in costs.

A recent analysis of 1993 national Medicare data reached similar conclusions (Welch, Wennberg, & Welch, 1996). It compared age- and sex-adjusted utilization rates to determine whether metropolitan statistical areas with higher rates of home health care also had lower hospital admission rates or lengths of stay. There was no evidence that home health care was substituting for hospital care or nursing home care. Home health care use was associated with higher rates of hospital admission. In addition, hospital stays preceded (by 30 or fewer days) only 22% of home health visits of the 160 million visits studied; thus, these visits probably served to ease hospital discharge. Nearly half (43%) of visits were not associated with an inpatient visit in the previous 6 months. The majority (61%) of visits were to enrollees who received home care for 6 months or longer. The use of home health care services geographically varied more than did the use of other categories of Medicare services; the state with the highest use had almost 10 times as many home health care visits as the state with the lowest use, suggesting a lack of consensus about the appropriate use of this care.

Two recent studies were more hopeful. One was a randomized trial of a home health care program for persons discharged from a hospital in Sweden. It found a statistically significant 20% cost reduction due to a smaller number of long-term hospital days by the home care group (Melin et al., 1993). Another study, this one of a home care program at a Veterans Administration (VA) hospital, reported cost reductions, although they were not statistically significant (Hughes et al., 1990, 1992).

Finally, a meta-analysis of 20 studies of home health care, not including the now more common programs that combine home care with other CBLTC programs, also found a small to moderate effect size of home care on the number of hospital days (Hughes et al., 1997). Positive effects were associated with nonrandomized designs, and information on costs was not available. This research group is now conducting a large multisite randomized trial of home care programs in the VA that include careful patient targeting, intensive efforts to control hospital admissions, and other procedures characteristic of the program at the single-site trial. Results from the multisite trial will be available in 1999.

Turning to the effect of home care on nursing home use, most studies reviewed show little evidence of impact, although the most recent study available for review has shown very promising results (Weissert, Lesnick, Musliner & Foley, 1997). There, in a statewide, capitated managed care program for Medicaid-eligible patients, CBLTC appeared to save 40% of the cost of nursing home care. One critical element may have been the very careful screening techniques to limit the client population to only those at high risk of nursing home long stay. State employees, rather than providers, performed eligibility assessments—an important departure from most studies. Eligibility for home care required that the patient be at risk for a nursing home stay of at least 3 months, not just nursing home entry. Another cost-limiting factor was a budget target for home care plans of only about one third of nursing home costs. Finally, we must note that the study employed a quasi-experimental design in which actual nursing home stays and costs were compared with those expected for such patients based on national data. Results might have differed if a randomized controlled trial had been used.

RESULTS FOR SUBGROUPS OF PATIENTS

Several studies examined whether the impact of CBLTC differed by the type of patient, because CBLTC programs serve heterogeneous populations, and an understanding of differential impact can form the basis for targeting these resources to those most likely to benefit. In contrast to the evidence on the overall effectiveness of CBLTC, evidence on the types of patients most likely to benefit is much more difficult to summarize and must be interpreted with extreme caution due to (1) problems and inconsistencies in the methods used by the studies to perform subgroup analyses, (2) small numbers of patients in most subgroups, (3) differences in the definition of subgroups across studies, (4) inconsistent results both within and across studies, (5) the large number of subgroup analyses increasing the likelihood that significant findings are due to chance, and (6) the study result that most subgroup analyses did not find groups that appeared to benefit more than others. Moreover, the types of patients discussed below are subgroups of patients already selected from the larger group referred to such programs who met study admission criteria. These admission criteria were based on earlier findings about those thought most likely to benefit from such programs.

Subgroup Results for Health Status Outcomes.   Findings suggest that younger, minimally disabled patients and those with social support may be more likely to benefit from CBLTC programs (Birnbaum et al., 1984; Katz et al., 1972; Blenkner, et al., 1970; Nielsen, 1972; Posman et al., 1964). In contrast, other studies found that less disabled patients had worse overall health and emotional health outcomes when placed in adult day health care programs (Eagle et al., 1991) and high-risk patients in CBLTC may be more likely to benefit in terms of survival (Grannemann et al., 1986).

Subgroup Results for Utilization and Cost Outcomes.   Several studies found evidence of reduced nursing home use and/or cost for some subgroups, although the findings are contradictory across studies. Patients at high risk for nursing home use—in a nursing home at or before the study began, on a nursing home wait list, meeting criteria found to predict placement (e.g., severe physical impairment or behavior problems)—were found to have lower nursing home use in some studies (Commonwealth of Massachusetts, 1975; Grannemann et al., 1986; Hedrick et al., 1993). On the other hand, higher-risk patients used more nursing home services in one model (Grannemann et al., 1986), while lower-risk patients used fewer nursing home services in some situations (Grannemann et al., 1986; Katz et al., 1972).

In terms of reduced hospital stays, certain types of patients appeared to benefit from these services: those who were over 75 and lived alone (Birnbaum et al., 1984), were terminally ill (in a meta-analysis by Hughes et al., 1997), were not severely disabled (Katz et al., 1972), had moderate unmet needs (Grannemann et al., 1986), had a good prognosis (Birnbaum et al., 1984), and were at high risk of institutionalization (Birnbaum et al., 1984).

The hopeful finding among terminally ill patients is at variance with a reanalysis of three subgroups of patients by Weissert, Lafata, Williams and Weissert (1997). They used data from the National Channeling Demonstration (Carcagno & Kemper, 1987) project to explore home care's effects on hospitalizations of three subgroups not analyzed by the original researchers. For the reanalysis, the authors hypothesized that home care would reduce hospitalizations resulting in death, nursing home placement, or evaluation without health status change. They speculated that home care is well equipped to alter these outcomes, as all three may involve some discretionary admissions possibly avoidable with the in-home support provided by home care. Results showed otherwise. There were no differences in these three types of hospitalization between the randomized treatment and control groups. The research group concluded that these three types of hospitalization probably deserve more specially focused preventive clinical effort.

Subgroup results from another randomized controlled trial, the Adult Day Health Care (ADHC) Evaluation study (Hedrick et al., 1993), may be instructive. This study, conducted in eight VA medical centers, found no subgroups that appeared to benefit in terms of health status. The study, however, did find one subgroup of patients who actually had significantly lower total costs when referred to ADHC: patients with 50% and greater service-connected disabilities (severe disabilities associated with military service). An analogous group in the civilian sector would be severely disabled patients who receive all health services at no cost and with few restrictions. The service-connected patients had significantly lower nursing home, clinic, home care, and pharmacy and lab costs when referred to ADHC. One could speculate that ADHC served a case management function for these patients who have easy access to care. Other groups had total costs of care that were not higher than those receiving customary care: patients with less than 50% service-connected disabilities, patients with multiple behavior problems, patients with high levels of impairment in physical function, and patients with a high risk of nursing home placement. This study also found that it would be prudent to avoid sending certain patients to ADHC because their costs of care were significantly higher than when assigned to customary care; these were patients with moderate or low levels of impairment in physical function and those with few behavior problems.

LESSONS FOR CLINICIANS

Clinicians have not had a clear sense of the specific positive outcomes that CBLTC should produce for a given patient nor the mix, amount, duration, or intensity of services needed to achieve benefits (Kemper, 1988). Nor have clinicians been very accurate in predicting adverse outcomes (Wan & Weissert, 1983). The result has been that many patients have been provided care to ameliorate risks that they did not actually face (e.g., long nursing home stays). Care plans authorized care that may have been more extensive and expensive than was necessary to achieve the limited benefits that CBLTC can actually produce (Kemper, 1988).

Clinicians need to improve their risk prediction to better target services to patients most likely to benefit. In particular, they should incorporate into their clinical judgments quantitative risk scores for hospitalization or long-stay nursing home use—not as a replacement for clinical decisions, but as one important factor. If the pattern of subgroup results described above were confirmed in future research, it would suggest that, to improve health status and possibly avoid hospital stays, CBLTC would need to target younger, healthier, less dependent, cognitively functional, socially supported patients. But to avoid nursing home stays and provide these services for the least additional cost over that of customary care, CBLTC would need to target older, extremely dependent, cognitively impaired, socially deprived patients with behavioral problems—that is, those at high risk of institutionalization. The essential lesson is to fit the care to the risks faced by individual patients.

Clinicians should also consider that, for many CBLTC patients, the costs of less care may equal those of more care. Clinicians should give their patients all the care they need, keeping in mind that in past studies, higher levels of care intensity, costliness, and duration have not improved financial outcomes (Weissert et al., 1988, 1989). As a general rule, patients are likely to receive the most benefits early in their episode of service use (Applebaum, Christianson, Harrigan, & Schore, 1988; Weissert, Wan, Livieratos, & Katz, 1980). If cuts have to be made to keep care costs under control, reductions in later stages or longer episodes are less likely to produce adverse effects than denying initial care to new patients.

Preventing unnecessary rehospitalization should be a constant concern, one that requires advanced planning and specific targeting of services to only those patients at risk for hospitalization. Aides or nurses are likely to call upon physicians to make quick decisions about hospitalizing CBLTC patients. Unless the physician has considered the likelihood of such an event and prepared for it, the usual practice will result in hospitalization. Yet in some cases, hospitalization can be avoided if the clinician has precise questions for the aide or nurse, an awareness of patient and family preferences for care, a sense of the aide's or nurse's reliability, and a judgment of whether the hospitalization is likely to actually benefit the particular patient. To avoid inappropriate hospitalizations, clinicians should counsel patients on the risks and benefits of hospitalized care. When continued independence appears doubtful, families and patients should be urged to visit nursing homes, make financial arrangements, and plan for an orderly transition to a nursing home without using the hospital as a staging area for decision-making (Weissert, Lafata, Williams, & Weissert, 1997).

LESSONS FOR MANAGERS AND POLICY MAKERS

Expecting most patients to substitute CBLTC for nursing home care is unrealistic. Most who use it will not be at high risk for nursing home use. As a group, home care patients are about 5 years younger than nursing home patients, and they have fewer risk factors for nursing home use. More home care patients are married, fewer have multiple dependencies in activities of daily living, and fewer suffer mental disorders. Managers and policymakers have been misled into believing that CBLTC saves substantial amounts of nursing home and hospital dollars, which wrongly suggests that CBLTC can be cost-effective while still spending relatively large amounts per patient. As a group, CBLTC patients are not likely to save much more than 15% of a year's nursing home costs even though some individual patients will save more and others will save less (Weissert et al., 1989). Many programs, expecting that a year of nursing CBLTC would be saved by every single home care patient, have had no budget constraint on CBLTC costs or caps set so high that they constrained spending to only the few most disabled patients in the demonstration (Carcagno & Kemper, 1987). Net costs will rise whenever CBLTC costs generated by keeping patients out of inpatient settings exceed savings on inpatient care. Since CBLTC is only minimally effective in avoiding inpatient care, CBLTC budgets must be low to avoid net cost increases.

Appropriate client selection and maintaining an adequate census are absolutely essential to achieving or even nearing cost-effectiveness. Demand estimates are likely to be unrealistically high (Weissert et al., 1990). Initial enrollment rates are unlikely to be sustained after pent-up demand is served. Cost-effectiveness of CBLTC is directly affected by the wording of eligibility criteria: Vague criteria tend to relax admission standards, producing a client population less likely to offset some of its cost by substituting CBLTC for other types of care. As enrollment rates drop and deaths and discharges erode the census, pressure will build to relax eligibility criteria. Vigilance is required to assure that minimum criteria are not allowed to slip and that the mix of patients is maintained.

Since clinicians are likely to err in the direction of providing care to patients at low risk rather than denying them care, managers must ensure that when a low-risk patient is admitted, the admitting clinician has a clear outcome goal for the patient, one that requires the level of CBLTC prescribed. If overall case mix complexity and severity decline over time, retraining of admitting teams may be necessary.

Several organizational arrangements help to control costs: placing multiple services under one management unit; associating CBLTC units with housing units (which also enhances demand); sharing staff and supplies; and allowing CBLTC units to be charged marginal, rather than average, costs for services they receive from larger units. Charging average costs invites cost-shifting from other cost centers that may be experiencing high costs due to falling inpatient census. Shifting average costs to CBLTC operations fails to take the opportunity to improve inpatient unit productivity by asking staff to assume CBLTC duties in addition to existing duties. Excessive staffing of the CBLTC unit (by unnecessarily assigning excess inpatient staff to CBLTC duties) will vitiate hopes for cost-effectiveness. Therapies and other services required only occasionally should be purchased rather than provided directly; experience shows that few CBLTC patients use such therapies, making it expensive to incorporate them into the CBLTC staff. Contracting for the entire CBLTC program may increase the potential for program targeting and cost-effective operations in some locations (Hedrick et al., 1993).

Managers should monitor care planners for variation in care plans for similar patients. Timely discharge from CBLTC should be part of care planning and review. Managers should also be alert that some patients will incur very high costs. For such patients, congregate settings may be more appropriate than CBLTC. Insurance should be maintained if the CBLTC program bears financial risk.

If cost-effectiveness can be achieved at all, it must come from avoiding hospital use, which has proved to be challenging for CBLTC programs. Managers can promote the quality of decision-making by helping to set up protocols to follow when a hospitalization is anticipated.

Policymakers can best facilitate cost-effective CBLTC by establishing budget caps that promote cost-effectiveness and by assisting management with demand studies, cost and utilization tracking software, and budget perspectives that acknowledge cost savings wherever they occur, not only when they accrue to specific organizational budgets. Autonomy in managing the CBLTC unit can protect it from demands to support staff that are inappropriate in terms of discipline, training, or interest in community-based care. The units also need the authority to not admit patients who have low likelihood of benefit but who are referred because of lack of other appropriate placements or inaccurate staff or patient/family expectations.

IMPLICATIONS FOR EVIDENCE-BASED PRACTICE

Community-based long-term care patients are a heterogeneous group. They require the same careful matching of treatment to diagnosed risk that typifies the evidence-based practicing physician's role in the rest of health care. Vague presumptions of nursing home or hospital risk and off-the-shelf care plans will not achieve optimal outcomes. Some patients require short-term postacute stabilization. Others risk acute flare-ups of chronic conditions and require aggressive disease management. A small group requires home-delivered high-tech procedures, which in the past were delivered only in inpatient settings. But most patients fall into none of these categories. They are lifers—patients who will be in such care for many years, avoiding such mundane risks as decline of function, breakdown of skin condition, decline of patient or family life satisfaction, or avoidance of hospitalizations precipitated by failure of the patient and family to come to grips with and prepare for inevitable nursing home placement or death. The hospital becomes a staging area for decisions that could have been made at home with proper advanced counseling. For these patients, appropriate outcomes are those that take advantage of CBLTC's full range of resources: aides familiar with the patient and family, their limitations and resources; nurses fully qualified to monitor vital signs and administer treatments; long-term physician relationships with the patient and family. CBLTC is ill equipped to alter health status. It is neither medical nor invasive, and it is rarely therapeutic. It is mostly supportive. What it can do, when properly managed by the physician, is alter how the patient, the family, and the physician respond to changes in health status. CBLTC is best equipped to monitor, help cope, and prepare for inevitable but unpredictable health status changes.

Hospitalization is best avoided by first quantitatively evaluating the risk of hospitalization, then among those at risk, evaluating probable underlying causes, such as hospitalization for nursing home placement decision-making, terminal care, failure of disease management in unstable patients, evaluation of health status change (which could have been done at home), and writing care plans calling for aggressive steps to prevent these specific hospitalizations.

Nursing home placement is best avoided by first quantifying the patient's risk of nursing home placement. If it is elevated, then again the underlying causes must be evaluated and a care plan written for interventions such as the installation of an emergency response system to reassure the patient and his or her family.

ADL decline is even less tractable. One important preventive action is to continue to exercise the function. Aides who are too willing to jump to the patient's assistance can quickly displace the patient's own ability to perform a function.

Avoiding declining life satisfaction in the patient or family seems to be a benefit that CBLTC can bestow on frail elderly patients. But there is little evidence to suggest the particular aspects of care that best produce improvements or at least slow the rate of decline. Minimalist levels of care may do as much good as more involved efforts.

The important rule of thumb in CBLTC is to recognize that most patients will show few benefits that are measurable as health status improvements. Care must be taken to subgroup patients into those for whom enhanced medical management will produce improvements versus those for whom care promises few benefits. Care should be allocated accordingly, more to those who face important tractable risks, less for those who are likely to benefit maximally from minimal treatment.

Managed care organizations are in an excellent position to make effective use of CBLTC. They are not bound by ill-conceived public policies that view CBLTC principally as a substitute for nursing home care. Hence they have the ability to adjust doses to the patient's risks and benefit potential. At a minimum, the Arizona Medicaid home care experience suggests that excessive, extended utilization can be avoided by separating postacute from long-term home care. Arizona incorporates postacute home care into its hospital per diem rate. Long-term home care is available only to patients who are likely to need at least 3 months of nursing home care. For the former, the goal is postacute stabilization and avoidance of hospital readmission. For the latter, the goal should be long-term, low-level maintenance in the community, probably best carried out by a subcontractor accustomed to marshaling family and community resources to develop and maintain a low-cost care plan.

REFERENCES

Applebaum, R. A., Chistianson, J. B., Harrigan, M., & Schore, J. (1988). The evaluation of the National Long-term Care Demonstration: The effect of channeling on mortality, functioning, and well-being. *Health Services Research, 23,* 143–159.

Benjamin, A. E. (1993). An historical perspective on home care policy. *Milbank Quarterly, 71,* 129.

Bergner, M., Hudson, L., Conrad, D., Patmont, C. M., McDonald, G. J., Perrin, E. B., & Gilson, B. S. (1988). The cost and efficacy of home care for patients with chronic lung disease. *Medical Care, 26,* 566–579.

Berkeley Planning Associates. (1987). *Evaluation of the ACCESS: Medicare long-term care demonstration projects.* Berkeley, CA: Author.

Birnbaum, H., Gaumer, G., Pratter, F., & Burke, R. (1984). *Nursing home without walls: Evaluation of the New York State long-term home health care program.* Cambridge, MA: Abt Associates.

Blenkner, M., Bloom, M., & Nielsen, M. (1971). A research and demonstration project of protective services. *Social Casework, 52,* 483–499.

Blenkner, M., Bloom, M., Nielsen, M., & Beggs, H. (1970). *Home aide service and the aged: A controlled study: Part 1. Design and findings. Part 2. The service program.* Cleveland: Benjamin Rose Institute.

Brown, T. E., Jr., Blackman, D. K., Learner, R. M., Witherspoon, M. B., & Saber, L. (1985). *South Carolina long-term care project: Report of findings.* Spartanburg: South Carolina State Health and Human Services Finance Commission.

Carcagno, G. J., & Kemper, P. (1987). An overview of the channeling demonstration and its evaluation. *Health Services Research, 23,* 3–21.

Commonwealth of Massachusetts (1975). *Home care: An alternative to institutionalization.* Boston: Commonwealth of Massachusetts, Department of Elder Affairs.

Eagle, D. J., Guyatt, G. H., Patterson, C., Turpie, I., Sackett, B., & Singer, J. (1991). Effectiveness of a geriatric day hospital. *Canadian Medical Association Journal, 144,* 699–704.

Gaumer, G. L., Birnbaum, H., Pratter, F., Burke, R., Franklin, S., & Ellingson-Otto, K. (1986). Impact of the New York long-term home health care program. *Medical Care, 24,* 641–653.

Grannemann, T. W., Grossman, J. B., & Dunstand, S. M. (1986). *Differential impacts among subgroups of channeling enrollees.* Princeton, NJ: Mathematica Policy Research, Enterprise Business Center.

Hanchett, E., & Torrens, P. R. (1967). A public health home nursing program for outpatients with heart disease. *Public Health Reports, 82,* 683–688.

Hedrick, S. C., Chapko, M. K., Ehreth, J. L., Rothman, M. L., Kelly, J. R., & Inui, T. S. (1993). Implications of the adult day health care evaluation study for program revision and research. *Medical Care, 31,* SS104–SS115.

Hedrick, S. C., Koepsell, T. D., & Inui, T. S. (1989). Meta-analysis of home care effects on mortality and nursing home placement. *Medical Care, 27,* 1015–1026.

Hedrick, S. C., Rothman, M. L., Chapko, M., Ehreth, J. L., Diehr, P., Inui, T. S., Connis, R. T., Grover, P. L., & Kelly, J. R. (1993). Summary and discussion of methods and results of the adult day health care evaluation. *Medical Care, 31,* SS94–SS103.

Hughes, S. L., Cordray, D. S., & Spiker V. A. (1984). Evaluation of a long-term home care program. *Medical Care, 22,* 640.

Hughes, S. L., Cummings, J., Weaver, F., Manheim, L., Braun, B., & Conrad, K. (1992). A randomized trial of the cost effectiveness of VA hospital-based home care for the terminally ill. *Health Services Research, 26,* 801–817.

Hughes, S. L., Cummings, J., Weaver, F., Manheim, L. M., Conrad, K. J., & Nash, K. (1990). A randomized trial of Veterans Administration home care for severely disabled veterans. *Medical Care, 28,* 135–145.

Hughes, S. L., Ulasevich, A., Weaver, F. M., Henderson, W., Manheim, L., Kubal, J.

D., & Bonarigo, F. (1997). The impact of home care on hospital days: A meta-analysis. *Health Services Research.* 32(4) 415–432.

Kane, R. L., Wales, J., Bernstein, L., Leibowitz, A., & Kaplan, S. (1984). A randomized controlled trial of hospice care. *Lancet,* (8382), 890–894.

Katz, S., Ford, A. B., Downs, T. D., Adams, M., & Rusby, D. I. (1972). *Effects of continued care: A study of chronic illness in the home* (DHEW Pub. No. HSM 73, 3010). Cleveland: Case Western Reserve University School of Medicine.

Kemper, P. (1988). The evaluation of the national long-term care demonstration: 10. Overview of the findings. *Health Services Research, 23,* 161–174.

Lawton, M. P., Brody, E. M., & Saperstein, A. R. (1989). A controlled study of respite service for caregivers of Alzheimer's patients. *Gerontologist, 29,* 8–16.

Maurer, J. M., Ross, N. L., & Bigos, Y. M. (1984). Final report and evaluation of the Florida Pentastar project. Tallahassee: Florida Department of Health and Rehabilitative Services.

Melin A., Hakansson S., & Bygren L. O. (1993). The cost-effectiveness of rehabilitation in the home: A study of Swedish elderly. *American Journal of Public Health, 83,* 356–362.

Mor, V., Greer, D. S., & Kastenbaum, R. (1988). *The hospice experiment.* Baltimore: Johns Hopkins University Press.

Nielsen, M., Blenkner, M., Bloom, M., Downs, & Beggs, H. (1972). Older persons after hospitalization: A controlled study of home aide service. *American Journal of Public Health, 62,* 1094–1101.

Oktay, J. S., & Volland, P. J. (1986). *Evaluating a support program for families of the frail elderly.* Paper presented at the annual meeting of the Gerontological Society of America, Chicago.

O'Rourke, B., Raisz, H., & Segal, J. (1982). Triage II: Coordinated delivery of services to the elderly (Vol.1–2). Plainville, CT: Triage.

Papsidero, J. A., Katz, S., Kroger, M. H., & Akpom, C. A. (1979). *Chance for change: Implications of a chronic disease module.* East Lansing: Michigan State University Press.

Petersen, M. D., & White, D. L. (1989). An information synthesis approach for reviewing literature. In M. D. Petersen & D. L. White (Eds.), *Health care of the elderly: An information sourcebook,* (pp. 26–36). Newbury Park: Sage Publications.

Pinkerton, A., & Hill, D. (1984). *Long-term care demonstration project of North San Diego County: Final report* (NTIS No. PB85-10391). San Diego: Allied Home Health Association.

Posman, H., Kogan, L. S., LeMat, A., & Dahlin, B. A. (1964). *Continuity in care for impaired older persons: Public health nursing in a geriatric rehabilitation maintenance program.* New York: Department of Public Affairs and Institute of Welfare Research, Community Service Society of New York.

Sainer, J. S., Brill, R. S., & Horowitz, A. (1984). *Delivery of medical and social services to the homebound elderly: A demonstration of intersystem coordination.* New York: New York City Department for the Aging.

Seidl, F. W., Applebaum, R., Austin, C., & Mahoney, K. (1983). *Delivering in-home services to the aged and disabled: The Wisconsin experiment.* Lexington MA: Lexington Books.

Selmanoff, E. D., Mitchell, R. U., Widlock, F. W., & Mossholder, M. A. (November,

1979). *Home care of geriatric patients by a health maintenance team.* Paper presented at the annual meeting of the American Public Health Association, New York.

Skellie, A., Favor, F., Tudor, C., & Strauss, R. (1982). *Alternative health services project: Final report.* Atlanta: Georgia Department of Medical Assistance.

Sklar, B. W., & Weiss, L. J. (1983). *Project OPEN (Organization Providing for Elderly Needs): Final report.* San Francisco: Mount Zion Hospital and Medical Center.

Wade, D. T., Langton-Hewer, R., Skilbeck, C. E., Bainton, D., & Burns-Cox, C. (1985). Controlled trial of a home-care service for acute stroke patients. *Lancet, 1,* 323–326.

Wan, T., & Weissert, W. (1983). Accuracy of prognostic judgments of elderly long-term care patients. *Archives of Gerontology and Geriatrics, 2,* 265–273.

Weissert, W. G. (1990). Strategies for reducing home care expenditures. *Generations* (Spring), 42–44.

Weissert, W. G., Cready, C. M., & Pawelak, J. E. (1988). The past and future of home-and community-based long-term care. *Milbank Quarterly, 66,* 309–388.

Weissert, W. G., Cready, C. M., & Pawelak, J. E. (1989). Home and community care: Three decades of findings. In M. D. Petersen & D. L. White (Eds.), *Health care of the elderly: An information source book* (pp. 39–126). Newbury Park: Sage Publications.

Weissert, W. G., Elston, J. M., Bolda, E. L., Zelman, W. N., Mutran, E., & Mangum, A. B. (1990). *Adult day care: Findings from a national survey.* Baltimore: Johns Hopkins University Press.

Weissert, W. G., & Hedrick, S. C. (1994). Lessons learned from research on effects of community-based long-term care. *Journal of the American Geriatrics Society, 42,* 348–353.

Weissert, W. G., Lafata, J. E., Williams, B., & Weissert, C. S. (1997). Toward a strategy for reducing potentially avoidable hospital admissions among home care clients. *Medical Care Research and Review, 54*(4), 439–455.

Weissert, W. G., Lesnick, T., Musliner, M., & Foley, K. (1997). Cost-savings from home- and community-based services: Arizona's capitated Medicaid long-term care program. *Journal of Health Politics, Policy and Law, 2*(6), 1329–1357.

Weissert, W. G., Wan, T., Livieratos, B., & Katz, S. (1980). Effects and costs of day-care services for the chronically ill: A randomized experiment. *Medical Care, 28,* 567–584.

Weissert, W. G., Wan, T. T. H., Livieratos, B., & Pellegrino, J. (1980). Cost-effectiveness of homemaker services for the chronically ill. *Inquiry, 17,* 230–243.

Welch, H. G., Wennberg, D. E., & Welch, W. P. (1996). The use of Medicare home health care services. *New England Journal of Medicine, 335,* 324–329.

Zawadski, R. T., Shen, J., Yordi, C., & Hansen, J. C. (1984). *On Lok's community care organization for dependent adults: A research and development project (1978–1983).* San Francisco: On Lok Senior Health Services.

Zimmer, J. G., Groth-Junker, A., & McCusker, J. (1985). A randomized controlled study of a home health care team. *American Journal of Public Health, 75,* 134–141.

13

Comprehensive Care of Older People With Alzheimer's Disease

Deirdre Johnston and Burton V. Reifler

INTRODUCTION

At least 1.8 million people in the United States have severe dementia, and an additional 1 million to 5 five million have mild-to-moderate dementia. The prevalence of dementia increases dramatically with age, affecting 25% or more of those over 85, the fastest growing segment of the population. People with dementia use some health and supportive services at higher rates than their nondemented age-matched counterparts (Philp et al., 1995; Souetre et al., 1995). Family costs, both direct and indirect, are substantial (Stommel, Colling, & Given, 1994). In the United States in 1991, 1.35 million cases of Alzheimer's disease accounted for an estimated $67.3 billion in total direct and indirect costs (Ernst & Hay, 1994).

The United States has few systems of care designed for dementia patients. Fragmentation of care and lack of community services accelerate the use of hospitals and nursing homes (Murphy & Banerjee, 1993). Whereas in the United Kingdom and Canada, comprehensive networks are evolving to serve the growing needs of the aging population, most physicians in the United States still practice in relative isolation. Medical education does not emphasize the integration of nonmedical care in addressing the problems encountered by frail older persons (see chapter 16). Awareness of psychosocial, functional, and environmental factors can be crucial in the care of the dementia patient. Caregiver burnout, for example, leads to premature admissions to hospitals and nursing homes. An effective alternative to inappropriate hospitalization and institutionalization may be the early identification of patients and caregivers at risk and the initiation of preventive, community-based services.

THE ROLE OF THE PRIMARY CARE PHYSICIAN

Families of Alzheimer's disease (AD) sufferers often turn to their primary care physicians for help. Initially, the physician must take time to diagnose the problem and address the family's understanding and expectations, as well as their grief. Some of the patient's lifelong habits may need to change. He or she may require help in managing several medications to avoid delirium, toxic interactions, and other complications, such as falls.

Unfortunately, physicians are more likely to order laboratory tests than to assess these patients' psychosocial or functional status (Fortinsky, Leighton, & Wasson, 1995). Due to the complexity of the issues involved in the care of AD, it is extremely difficult for physicians working alone to provide adequate care. The team model offers potentially effective ways of providing care to this population (Williams, Williams, Zimmer, Hall, & Podgorski, 1987).

Often the primary care physician functions as a gatekeeper to formal health care services and as a manager in guiding resource use and team function, all while continuing to provide medical care to a patient whose susceptibility to infections, falls, drug toxicity, malnutrition, and other medical problems increases as the disease advances. In many cases, this role includes the prescription of psychoactive medications for depression or paranoid symptoms. Although behavioral and psychiatric symptoms are risk factors for institutionalization (Steele, Rovner, Chase, & Folstein, 1990), counseling and support of caregivers of dementia sufferers have been shown to lengthen the time that the AD patient can remain home (Mittelman, Ferris, Shulman, Steinberg, & Levin, 1996). Skillful management of these behavioral symptoms, including insomnia, often alleviates the patient's and the family caregivers' distress. In the nursing home, the patient continues to need medical attention as the illness progresses and as the symptoms fluctuate according to the stage of the disease and the presence of intercurrent illnesses. There the physician supports the staff in assessing and managing behavioral problems.

The patient and family usually needs help in coping with the progression of the disease. The family needs to prepare to take charge of legal and financial affairs. Subsequent discussions must address driving, the use of firearms, and other preventive and emotionally charged subjects. Caregivers in many communities have established Alzheimer's support groups (McCarty, 1992), to which primary care physicians may refer their patients. Additionally, patients and families are able to optimize their use of both formal and informal services when they better understand the illness—through educational material, encouragement to ask questions, and help with planning for the future. Information on coping techniques, support groups, and similar resources enhances their sense of autonomy and may allow the patient to maintain a more satisfactory quality of life at home rather than in a care facility, particularly in the early stages of the illness (Mittelman et al., 1996).

With the emergence of new pharmacotherapy for AD, the physician may soon be able to delay the inevitable cognitive decline. The medications available now are the anticholinesterase agents tacrine and donepezil; several others are under study. Preventing deterioration in cognitive function has been projected to reduce substantially the costs of care in patients with moderate-to-severe Alzheimer's disease (Ernst, Hay, Fenn, Tinklenberg, & Yesavage, 1997).

The physician's role also includes attention to end-of-life issues. Very high health care costs (and poor quality of life) are experienced in the final days and weeks of life, often the result of heroic efforts to prevent death. Early planning with the patient and family regarding the patient's wishes (advance directives) may help increase quality of life, control over the events of the last days, and chances of dying with dignity.

SYSTEMS OF CARE

New systems of care are emerging that may improve quality of life and continuity of care. The team care management model designates one team member to plan care and to coordinate responses to the patient's changing needs as the disease progresses, allowing the patient to obtain necessary services in a timely manner and minimizing the need for urgent services. The emergence of managed care offers new opportunities for financing such coordinated approaches.

Most individuals with AD want to remain at home, a desire generally supported by their families. Institutionalization becomes more likely when the caregiver becomes exhausted or ill (Brown, Potter, & Foster, 1990) or when the patient has a hospital admission or becomes unmanageable at home (Thienhaus, Rowe, Woellert, & Hillard, 1988). Depressive symptoms are common among primary caregivers of AD sufferers (Mohide & Streiner, 1993). As the patient becomes more dependent on the caregiver, the caregiver often experiences the stress of isolation and a pressing need for periodic breaks from care duties. Support groups (for the caregiver) and adult day care programs and brief use of nursing homes (for the patient) all offer respite to the caregiver (Feinberg & Kelly, 1995).

Adult Day Centers

Adult day centers offer comprehensive, community-based programs for individuals with AD. Two large national demonstration programs of adult day centers, the Dementia Care and Respite Services Program (1988–1992) and Partners in Caregiving (1992–1997), have provided important insights into the feasibility of such programs (Cox & Reifler, 1994; Reifler et al., 1997). In one, the participants had an average of 4.2 medical problems, 3.8 impairments in activities of daily living (ADL), 8.8 behavior problems, and 13.4 on the Mini-Mental State Status Examination (possible range 0–30), thus confirming that these centers care for people with serious physical and mental disabilities, including dementia (Sherrill, Reifler, & Henry, 1994). They offer a range of activities such as exercise, crafts, music, and bathing. Some follow a medical model, while others follow a social model. The availability of health monitoring, usually by a nurse on the premises, distinguishes the medical model from the social one; other programming is common to both models.

In recent years, adult day centers have expanded their hours to meet better the needs of working caregivers; they have begun to operate on evenings and weekends as well. Many centers now offer activity tracks tailored to individuals with similar degrees of cognitive and functional impairment. For example, mildly impaired participants might spend more of their day occupied with verbal activities and crafts, while more impaired participants would be engaged with physical movement and slow-paced socialization. Music has application across the entire spectrum of dementia. Compared with nursing homes, adult day centers are less expensive (often about half the daily cost), more amenable to serving the patient and family for the number of days they want, and more reflective of a normal life in that the patient leaves home in the morning and returns at night.

But are adult day centers financially viable? Findings from the demonstration programs mentioned above show that they can be, as 21% (10/48) of the centers in Partners in Caregiving were fully self-supporting. Overall, the centers met an average of 83% of their expenses through fee-for-service revenue (usually a combination of self-pay and Medicaid), with the balance coming from in-kind support and local philanthropy. Day centers have been shown to reduce caregiver burden (Stephens, 1996), a particularly important attribute in light of the enormous difficulties involved in caring for people with AD.

Given the success of adult day centers, it is not surprising that their number has increased from only a handful 20 years ago to more than 4,000 in the United States in 1997 ("Adult Day Care," 1996), but this is still well short of the projected national need of 10,000 (Reifler, 1992).

Group Living

New approaches to residential care are also being tested. In Sweden, where 18% of the population is over 65, demented persons increasingly live in government-subsidized group homes, which reduce acute hospital use and cost less than nursing home care for healthy ambulatory demented patients (Wimo, Wallin, Lundgren, & Ronnback, 1991). Reports indicate that, compared to nursing homes, these units preserve more functioning (Kihlgren, 1992) by avoiding anxiety, maintaining orientation, and offering more opportunities for social interaction and involvement in normal daily activities. A 4-year follow-up study of 16 patients with dementia in group living units suggested that most of them had avoided institutional care for considerably longer than would have been possible at home. The main reason for institutionalization was aggression (Wimo, Asplund, Mattson, Adolfsson, & Lundgren, 1995). Multilevel residential programs are now available in many locations, offering independent living, assisted living, and nursing home care according to individuals' needs. Some offer dementia special care units.

The Dementia Special Care Unit (DSCU)

Adopting a palliative care philosophy, many long-term care institutions have developed DSCUs to provide supportive care to persons with AD who develop functional dependency or unsafe behaviors. When AD progresses such that significant physical care is required or ambulation is difficult, the patient may move to a DSCU. Advanced planning is emphasized and medical treatment is conservative and palliative, with attention to quality of life and comfort taking priority over life-prolonging interventions. In support of these goals, a 2-year prospective cohort study comparing a DSCU with a traditional long-term care facility found that DSCU patients exhibited less overall discomfort while having a higher mortality rate than the patients in traditional long-term care (Volicer et al., 1994).

In an effort to maximize patient comfort, DSCUs often employ environmental modification to prevent dangerous complications of dementia-induced behaviors. For example, the problem of patient wandering can be effectively controlled through a circular floor plan or by the use of visual barriers over hallway exits. One study demonstrated that simply covering the doorknob of an exit with a cloth was sufficient to stop all patient exits (Namazi, Rosner, & Calkins, 1989). Specially designed chairs and positioning devices can likewise obviate the need for restraint while maintaining the patient's comfort and dignity. Data from the Health Care Finance Administration (HCFA) Multi-state Case Mix and Quality Demonstration Project (MCMQDP) showed that fewer patients in DSCU's were physically restrained compared to traditional long-term care (TLTC); however, the

DSCU patients were more likely to be "chemically restrained," meaning that they were receiving antipsychotic, antianxiety, or hypnotic medications (Mehr & Fries, 1995).

It appears that it costs less to care for demented patients in a DSCU than in TLTC. A comparison of the two models showed that, although resource use (staff time and wages) was approximately the same for the two models (Mehr & Fries, 1995), savings are achieved in DSCUs through lower use of medications, laboratory services, and acute care facilities. One study showed that DSCU costs were approximately one eighth those of TLTC costs over a 3-month period; the bulk of these savings was achieved through dramatically lower use of acute care by the DSCU group (Volicer et al., 1994).

Numerous anecdotes would suggest that DSCU care results in improved patient functioning; however, the largest objective study to date does not support this notion. Using data from the MCMQDP, investigators measured functional decline in three groups of long-term care residents: 1,228 in DSCUs, 5,904 receiving TLTC within a facility that contained a DSCU, and 7,205 TLTC residents in non-DSCU facilities. The three groups exhibited the same rate of decline in nine functional outcomes over a 1-year period (Phillips et al., 1997).

There is considerable variation in the way DSCUs are organized and operated. Consequently, it is difficult to generalize the findings of a few studies to all care rendered in DSCUs. In general, however, DSCUs appear to be less costly than TLTC units for dementia. DSCU patients and caregivers may experience benefits of increased comfort and satisfaction with care, although mortality rates may be higher due to the palliative philosophy of DSCU care. DSCUs do not appear to slow the functional decline seen in patients afflicted with dementia.

Comprehensive Community-based Care

Systems that have been developed to provide comprehensive care to community-dwelling patients include the federal Program for All-inclusive Care for the Elderly and the Social Health Maintenance Organizations (discussed in chapter 16). Although neither has been designed specifically for the challenges of AD, both provide services that benefit AD patients. The Social Health Maintenance Organizations are currently developing systems for identifying and meeting the needs of at-risk patients, a goal that includes dementia sufferers. In one study, the use of an intense case management approach to the care of community-dwelling, chronically ill patients was most efficient for those patients who suffered from dementia, with apparent cost savings, but no difference in other health- or function-related outcomes (Zimmer, Eggert, & Chiverton, 1990).

The Alzheimer's Demonstration Project (ADP) was an HCFA-support-ed demonstration project in eight communities designed to increase the availability of supportive services for patients with AD and their family caregivers. The foundation of the program was case management provided with two different intensities in different communities (low intensity, with a 1:100 case manager-to-client ratio and a low cap on expenditures; and high intensity, with a 1:30 case manager-to-client ratio and a high cap on expenditures). In both models, HCFA paid for a wide range of supportive services, with 20% coinsurance for all but Medicaid beneficiaries. The pro-gram randomized patients in each community to receive either case man-agement or usual care.

Patients and caregivers randomized to the case management group received significantly more supportive services such as adult day care and homemaker, chore, and companion services than did the control patients. The early results suggested that the ADP intervention reduced the unmet needs of the clients and their caregivers but did not reduce nursing home admissions. The final results have not been published yet. Effective case management requires that effective medical and community services be available, which can be a problem if community providers are neither trained nor experienced in the complex management issues associated with AD (Baxter, 1997).

ELECTRONIC COMMUNICATION

As we enter a new millennium, emerging technologies may enable demen-tia sufferers and their caregivers to access care and support in novel ways. Caregivers who feel unable to leave demented loved ones alone can engage in social interactions and exchanges of information with similar caregivers over the Internet. Several Web sites provide information about the disease, available resources, and online caregiver support groups: http://www.mailbase.uk/lists/candid-dementia, http://werple.mira.net.au/~dhs/ad.html, and http://pw2.netcom/~lehdoll/eldercareCHAT.html. Additionally, electronic telecommunications systems that connect through patients' television sets may lead to additional support for patients and caregivers (Lindberg, 1997). Research is now evaluating new ways of pro-viding both primary and consultative care to demented people at remote locations, including nursing homes (Jones, 1996).

SUMMARY

As the population ages, the prevalence of AD and other dementias will continue to increase. The primary physician, increasingly practicing as a member of a team, will help to guide the dementia sufferer and his or her family to appropriate care. The physician needs to be informed about existing and new dementia-oriented clinical programs and community resources. Much more research is needed to optimize our ability to treat Alzheimer's disease and other dementing illnesses—through medications, lay and professional education, support for family caregivers, and organization of community and institutional care.

REFERENCES

Adult day care experienced tremendous growth in 17 years. (1996, December). *Adult Day Care Letter*, pp. 1–21.

Baxter, E. (1997). Patients, caregivers, and managing care. *Geriatrics, 52* (Supp. 2), 548–549.

Branch, L. G., Coulam, R. F., & Zimmerman, Y. A. (1995). The PACE evaluation: Initial findings. *Gerontologist, 35,* 349–359.

Brown, L. J., Potter, J. F., & Foster, B. G. (1990). Caregiver burden should be evaluated during geriatric assessment. *Journal of the American Geriatrics Society, 38,* 455–460.

Cox, N. J., & Reifler, B. V. (1994). Dementia care and respite services program. *Alzheimer's and Associated Disorders,* 8(Supp. 3), 113–121.

Ernst, R. L., & Hay, J. W. (1994). The United States economic and social costs of Alzheimer's disease revisited. *American Journal of Public Health, 84,* 1261–1264.

Ernst, R. L., Hay, J. W., Fenn, C., Tinklenberg, J., & Yesavage, J. A. (1997). Cognitive function and the costs of Alzheimer's disease. *Archives of Neurology, 54,* 687–693.

Feinberg, L. F., & Kelly, K. A. (1995). A well-deserved break: Respite programs offered by California's statewide system of caregiver resource center. *Gerontologist, 35,* 701–706.

Fortinsky, F. H., Leighton, A., & Wasson, J. H. (1995). Primary care physicians' diagnostic management, and referral practices for older persons and families affected by dementia. *Research on Aging, 17,* 124–148.

Jones, B. N. (1996). Telemedicine and long-term care. *Nursing Home Economics, 3,* 17–19.

Kihlgren, M. (1992). Long-term influences on demented patients in different caring milieus, a collective living unit and a nursing home: A descriptive study. *Dementia, 3,* 342–349.

Lindberg, C. C. (1997). Implementation of in-home telemedicine in rural Kansas: Answering an elderly patient's needs. *Journal of the American Medical Informatics Association, 4,* 14–17.

McCarty, P. A. (1992). Health care policy and the Alzheimer's patient: A policy assessment of changes in the mental health system's response to victims of dementing illness. *Journal of Geriatric Psychiatry, 25,* 169–181.

Mehr, D. R., & Fries, B. E. (1995). Resource use on Alzheimer's special care units. *Gerontologist, 35,* 179–184.

Mittelman, M., Ferris, S., Shulman, E., Steinberg, G., & Levin, B. (1996). A family intervention to delay nursing home placement of patients with Alzheimer disease: A randomized controlled trial. *Journal of the American Medical Association, 276,* 1725–1731.

Mohide, E. A., & Streiner, D. L. (1993). Depression in caregivers of impaired elderly family members. In P. Cappelliez & R. Flynn (Eds.), *Depression and the social environment: Research and intervention in neglected populations* (pp. 289–331). Montreal: McGill-McQueen's University Press.

Murphy, E., & Banerjee, S. (1993). The organization of old-age psychiatry services. *Reviews in Clinical Gerontology, 3,* 367–378.

Namazi, K. H., Rosner, T. T., & Calkins, M. P. (1989). Visual barriers to prevent ambulatory Alzheimer's patients from exiting through an emergency door. *Gerontologist, 29,* 699–702.

Phillips, C. D., Sloane P. D., Hawes, C., Koch, G., Han, J., Spry, K., Dunteman, G., & Williams, R. L. (1997). Effects of residence in Alzheimer disease special care units on functional outcomes. *Journal of the American Medical Association, 278,* 1340–1344.

Philp, I., McKee, K. J., Meldrum, P., Ballinger, B. R., Gilhooly, M. L. M., Gordon, D. S., Mutch, W. J., & Whittick, J. E. (1995). Community care for demented and non-demented elderly people: A comparison study of financial burden, service use, and unmet needs in family supporters. *British Medical Journal, 310,* 1503–1506.

Reifler, B. V. (1992). Making something good out of something bad. *Respite Report* 4, 3.

Reifler, B. V., Henry, R. S., Fushing J., Yates, K., Cox, N. S., Bradham, D. D., & McFarlane, M. (1997). Financial performance among adult day centers. *Journal of the American Geriatrics Society, 45,* 146–153.

Sherrill, K. A., Reifler, B. V., & Henry, R. S. (1994). Respite care for dementia caregivers: Findings from the Robert Wood Johnson Foundation Projects. In E. Light, G. Niederehe, & B. D. Lebowitz (Eds.), *Stress effects of family caregivers of Alzheimer's patients: Research and interventions* (pp. 222–223). New York: Springer.

Souetre, E. J., Qing, W., Vigoureux, I., Dartigues, J.-F., Lozet, H., Lacomblez, L., & Derouesne, C. (1995). Economic analysis of Alzheimer's disease in outpatients: Impact of symptom severity. *International Psychogeriatrics, 7,* 115–122.

Steele, C., Rovner, B., Chase, G., & Folstein, M. (1990). Psychiatric symptoms and nursing home placement of patients with Alzheimer's disease. *American Journal of Psychiatry, 147,* 1049–1051.

Stephens, M. A. P. (1996). *Day care and family strain: Testing the effects of intervention.* Paper presented at the meeting of the Gerontological Society of America. November, Washington, DC.

Stommel, J., Colling, C. E., & Given, B. A. (1994). The costs of family contributions to the care of persons with dementia. *Gerontologist, 34,* 199–205.

Thienhaus, O. J., Rowe, C., Woellert, P., & Hillard, J. R. (1988). Geropsychiatric emergency services: Utilization and outcome predictors. *Hospital and Community Psychiatry, 39,* 1301–1305.

Volicer, L., Collard, A., Hurley, A., Bishop, C., Kern, K., & Karon, S. (1994). Impact of special care unit for patients with advanced Alzheimer's disease on patients' discomfort and costs. *Journal of the American Geriatrics Society, 42,* 597–603.

Williams, M., Williams T., Zimmer, J., Hall, W., & Podgorski, C. (1987). How does the team approach to out-patient geriatric evaluation compare with traditional care? A report of a randomized controlled trial. *Journal of the American Geriatrics Society, 35,* 1071–1078.

Wimo, A., Asplund, K., Mattson, B., Adolfsson, R., & Lundgren, K. (1995). Patients with dementia in group living: Experiences 4 years after admission. *International Psychogeriatrics, 7,* 123–127.

Wimo, A., Wallin, J. O., Lundgren, K., & Ronnback, E. (1991). Group living: An alternative for dementia patients. *International Journal of Geriatric Psychiatry, 6,* 21–29.

Zimmer, J. G., Eggert, G. M., & Chiverton, P. (1990). Individual versus team case management in optimizing community care for chronically ill patients with dementia. *Journal of Aging and Health, 2,* 357–372.

14

Long-Term Care in the Nursing Home

John F. Schnelle and David B. Reuben

INTRODUCTION

Currently, more than 20,000 licensed nursing homes (NHs) care for approximately 1.5 million residents in the United States (Strahan, 1997). These statistics assuredly will increase for a variety of reasons. First, population growth, increased longevity, and the continued lack of integrated chronic care networks will dramatically increase the number of functionally dependent older people. Among those age 65 years in 1990, approximately 43% will enter an NH at some time. Although many will be admitted for short stays, 55% of those admitted may stay for at least 1 year, and 21% may stay 5 years or longer (Kemper & Murtaugh, 1991). Moreover, the most rapidly growing segment of the older population is the group of persons 85 years of age or older; approximately 25% of this age group is institutionalized, the highest rate among all age groups (American Association of Retired Persons, 1995; Bureau of the Census, 1995). Accordingly, the Department of Health and Human Services (1991) predicts that the number of Americans residing in NHs will rise from 1.6 million in 1990 to 5.3 million in 2030. Several potential developments may attenuate this steep growth, including the improved organization and effectiveness of home health care and integrated chronic care networks and the development of preventive interventions that postpone the onset of chronic diseases.

However, despite uncertainty about how much the NH population will grow, NHs indubitably will continue to be a vital and expensive part of any chronic care network. In this chapter, we describe the organization and barriers to change of current NH care, then discuss three major forces that could shape the quality and structure of future NH care:

1. the impact of regulatory system innovation on the processes of assessment and care planning
2. the effects of practice guidelines
3. the potential effects of managed care

ORGANIZATION OF NURSING HOME CARE AND BARRIERS TO IMPROVEMENT

The overall purpose of this chapter is to describe how the forces listed above may change NH care in the future. As background, the reader needs a basic understanding of the structure and functions of current NHs. Accordingly, we begin by describing the roles of the NH staff, including problems with their organization, training, and management. Our discussion emphasizes staff who are most relevant to the direct care of long-term residents. We do not address subacute (transitional) care, a major new segment of the NH operations that is described in detail in chapter 8. We also do not address models for "reengineering" the roles of ancillary NH staff (e.g., housekeeping and food services), as information about such models is scarce.

Nursing aides provide 90% of the daily care in NHs (Mercer, Heacock, & Beck, 1993). Yet despite the importance of the nursing aide, little attention has focused on how to perform the nursing aide's job. For example, most homes assign 8 to 10 residents to each aide on the day shift and 12 to 15 residents to each aide on the evening shift. These job ratios stem from tradition and reimbursement realities rather than from formal analyses of what is needed. Moreover, scant knowledge exists about how to best organize aides' tasks to maximize productivity. Finally, NHs typically pay aides minimum wages and provide poor or perfunctory on-site training. Urgently needed are effective training models designed for aides who are poorly educated and who, in many urban areas, speak different languages and have different cultural norms than the residents for whom they provide care. Given the importance of the nursing aide job, it seems unlikely that care will improve significantly until more attention centers on fundamental issues concerning job design, wages, and training.

Aides receive direct supervision from "floor nurses," who themselves often possess less than 1 year of formal training. In most NHs, floor nurses work at nursing stations where they spend most of their time charting care activities and dispensing medicines. Typically, one floor nurse supervises five to six aides in caring for 50 residents. Few studies have examined the managerial skills of floor nurses.

The nursing aides and floor nurses receive supervision from a director of nurses and, depending on the size of the home, from several assistant directors or treatment nurses who are usually registered nurses. These professional nurses spend most of their time planning patient care and documenting that care meets regulatory standards; they rarely have time to provide direct care (Kane & Kane, 1987).

The high turnover of staff at all levels and the deficits in their knowledge of effective management for clinical problems are two additional barriers to improvements (Schnelle, Cruise, Rahman, & Ouslander, 1998). The example of a large program designed to improve incontinence care illustrates the importance of the turnover problem (Schnelle, McNees, Crooks, & Ouslander, 1995). The program provided nurses and aides in nine NHs with skills in patient care and quality management. One year after training, however, only one nurse remained in the same position as when training had begun.

Partially as a result of such turnover, the NH workforce lacks knowledge about many of the most common health problems of NH residents (e.g., physical disability and cognitive impairment). As a result, time efficiency often drives care routines, creating practices that foster dependency. Diapering and changing linens is more time-efficient, for example, than encouraging a resident to use the toilet regularly (Schnelle, Sowell, Hu, & Traughber, 1988).

A variety of other professionals and paraprofessionals administer social services, activities, and rehabilitation therapies (e.g., physical and occupational therapy) to NH residents. Although these services may improve the quality of life for NH residents, existing research data show that these therapies have limited effectiveness. For example, two studies that evaluated physical therapy in chronic long-term NH residents reported only very modest benefits (Chiodo, Gerety, Mulrow, Rhodes, & Tuley, 1992; Molloy & Richardson, 1988). Another study questions the effectiveness of the physical therapy model in which residents receive therapy for a limited period (e.g., 20 to 30 days), then return to usual nursing home care (Schnelle, MacRae, Ouslander, Simmons, & Nitta, 1995). Similarly, social service and activity therapists might play important roles in treating symptoms of depression, which are prevalent among NH residents (Abrams, Teresi, & Butin, 1992; Rovner et al., 1991), but the evidence does not suggest that they do so effectively, or even that depressive symptoms are adequately detected among NH residents (Rovner & Katz, 1994). Given the high cost of such therapies, evaluation of the cost-effectiveness seems warranted and may lead to fundamental changes in their use in the future.

Each NH has a medical director, usually a physician with a full-time medical practice elsewhere. This ill-defined role includes overseeing the quality of medical care at the NH and signing forms necessary for regulation and reimbursement. It is unusual, however, for medical directors to attempt proactively to affect medical quality (Dimant, 1991; Schnelle, 1995).

The absence of good information systems and practice guidelines, coupled with insufficient training in quality management principles and geriatrics, restricts the effectiveness of most medical directors.

The remainder of this chapter describes efforts to improve the clinical care in NHs. We argue that the effectiveness of these efforts will fall short unless the organizational issues described above also receive attention.

FORCES SHAPING QUALITY AND CHANGE IN NURSING HOME CARE

Regulatory Efforts to Improve Nursing Home Care: The MDS

Medical and lay literature in the 1980s documented the poor quality of care provided by many NHs. In 1986 the Institute of Medicine (IOM) issued a report offering numerous suggestions on how to improve NH care (Federal Register, 1991). The following year the Health Care Financing Administration (HCFA) generated new rules for licensed nursing facilities (contained in Omnibus Budget Reconciliation Act (OBRA) 1987) that incorporated many of the suggestions in the IOM report. These regulations mandated two new systems for assessing the status of NH residents: the Minimum Data Set (MDS) and a set of the Resident Assessment Protocols (RAPs) (Morris et al., 1991).

All NHs participating in the Medicare and Medicaid programs implemented the MDS/RAP system in 1991. The staff of these NHs periodically gather the data required by the MDS and use it to plan individualized care according to algorithms contained in the RAPs. The MDS covers a wide variety of functional domains (e.g., continence and physical abilities) and triggers more thorough assessments and actions (RAP) when a resident exhibits common problems, such as cognitive loss, incontinence, and pressure ulcers. The staff complete the MDS quarterly.

Survey teams from state regulatory agencies, which are responsible for ensuring the quality of NH care, visit all NHs annually to see that they are using the MDS according to regulatory standards. The survey teams also interview residents and attempt to observe care. However, the brief 2-to-3-day duration of the site visits limits the survey teams' capacity to assess care routines directly. Surveyors have not devised satisfactory methods to unobtrusively observe care interview representative residents who are capable of giving accurate information (Simmons et al., 1997).

The entire system, which emphasizes written assessment, consumes significant amounts of nursing time, but it does not address organizational and staffing barriers to improving NH care. In response to these regulations, many NHs have hired special nurses specifically to perform the tasks required by the MDS. This practice has generated suspicion that the MDS/RAP system is being subverted into a paper compliance program. Supporting this view, researchers have discerned two care processes—toileting and restraint release—that appear to be conducted more consistently in written care plans than in observed practice (Schnelle, Ouslander, & Cruise, 1997). The degree to which the MDS has truly changed the overall care provided as opposed to the care plans written is uncertain.

More optimistically, a recent series of quasi-experimental evaluations concluded that the MDS system has produced important changes in the processes and outcomes of NH care (Fries et al., 1997; Mor et al., 1997; Phillips et al., 1997). Before the full implementation of the MDS system, the investigators used the MDS assessment to track the prevalence of specific conditions (e.g., dehydration) and functional limitations during a 6-month period. They then conducted a second 6-month evaluation several years later after all NHs had implemented the MDS, comparing the outcomes in the pre-MDS and post-MDS periods. The authors reported reductions in hospitalization, use of urinary catheters, and rates of decline in cognitive and ADL functioning. They cited better written care planning as one reason for the improvements.

In summary, the MDS/RAP program has attempted to improve quality by providing information to providers and by motivating its use through a regulatory system. Although evidence suggests that this strategy has been at least partially successful, it is not yet clear how NHs have reallocated resources and changed their processes of care. Future evaluations of the MDS system should address the following questions:

1. How do NHs consistently implement new care processes despite high staff turnover in NHs? In particular, how do NHs train their nursing aides to use the MDS/RAP system in spite of the pervasive problems with language barriers, low educational levels, and high turnover rates?
2. How do providers, from physicians to aides, use the assessment data in their daily practices? Do residents actually receive more appropriate care?
3. Which specific practices produce better outcomes? The identification of effective, innovative care processes could lead to practice guidelines for care in all NHs.

Practice Guidelines

The practice guideline concept evolved at least partially in response to documented variability in how providers manage clinical problems. To improve quality and potentially reduce costs, practice guidelines aim to reduce this variability by providing advice on how to best assess and treat selected clinical problems. The U.S. Agency for Health Care Policy and Research (AHCPR) wrote the first guidelines for NH care—for urinary incontinence, pressure sore prevention, depression, and heart failure (Panel for Depression Guidelines, 1993; Panel for Heart Failure Evaluation and Care of Patients with Left-Ventricular Systolic Dysfunction, 1994; Panel for the Prediction and Prevention of Pressure Ulcers in Adults Guidelines, 1992; Panel for Urinary Incontinence in Adult Guidelines, 1996). More recently, other professional groups have assumed responsibility for developing and disseminating guidelines. The American Medical Directors Association (AMDA) has now taken the lead in developing practice guidelines specifically for NHs.

Guidelines generally take the form of algorithms that describe assessment actions and corresponding treatment options. They evolve from summaries of the state-of-the-art knowledge about common clinical problems. Many guidelines, however, lack the support of rigorous studies, recommending actions on the basis of expert consensus. Unfortunately, we do not know whether NHs actually use the current guidelines, much less whether the care prescribed in most guidelines is effective.

Many guidelines do not consider issues that are crucial to long-term care, perhaps contributing to their low usage in NHs (Schnelle et al., submitted). For example, they rarely address the logistics of providing interventions to residents. Also, the developers typically disseminate guidelines to NH professionals (e.g., medical directors, administrators, and nurses) through the mail and at training sessions at professional meetings. This assumes that those professionals will somehow educate other staff who are responsible for direct care in the NH. How such education might occur, who would pay for it, or even what its components might be is not specified.

In recognition of the implementation difficulties associated with multiple care providers, the AMDA is expanding its guideline development efforts from a clinical emphasis to also consider methods of dissemination, costs, and applicability to NH care. If guidelines are to overcome the organizational barriers to changing practice patterns in NHs, they must address three questions:

1. Which residents are likely to respond to treatment, and when should treatment be discontinued?
2. How much does the intervention cost in comparison to usual care, and who benefits from any cost reduction?
3. What techniques are available to facilitate the consistent implementation of the interventions described in the practice guidelines?

We now discuss each of these implementation issues in greater detail.

Long-term care residents with common problems (e.g., incontinence) usually suffer from a wide range of comorbidities. Because of them, residents show a wide range of responsiveness to protocols that address only one problem and are silent about the complicating effects of the others (Tinetti, Inouye, Gill, & Doucette, 1995). Therefore, NHs need effective methods to identify residents who will likely benefit from guideline-driven care. Without targeting criteria, providers may spend their limited resources providing interventions for many residents to whom certain guidelines are not relevant.

Guidance exists for targeting residents for incontinence treatment and for developing rules for stopping such treatment (Ouslander et al., 1995; Schnelle et al., 1993). If such targeting and stopping protocols do not accompany other guidelines, however, NH providers will have great difficulty implementing them, even if they are motivated to do so.

No practice guideline developed to date has estimated the costs an NH would incur for its implementation. Uncertainty about costs reduces NHs' motivation to start and maintain the implementation process, particularly if costs are likely to increase as a result. NHs often implement only guidelines that they expect to "save" money.

Many guidelines do indeed imply that their implementation will result in "savings." For example, the AHCPR incontinence guideline reports that complications of urinary incontinence cost approximately $3 billion annually, and it implies that successful treatment of incontinence would reduce these costs (Panel for Urinary Incontinence in Adult Guidelines, 1996). Unfortunately, this argument ignores the current mechanisms of NH reimbursement. Even if the optimistic cost-saving projections prove to be true, the NHs, which must pay the training and labor costs of implementing the incontinence interventions, would not be the primary beneficiaries. Instead, the primary beneficiaries would be third-party payers, such as Medicare, that pay for hospitalizations due to urinary tract infections and other problems related to urinary incontinence. Currently, no method exists for third-party payers to either share these savings or reimburse NHs for reducing the acute care costs of incontinence or any other problem. Integrating NHs into capitated provider networks may help solve this inequitable reimbursement situation. We discuss this type of solution in the Managed Care section of this chapter.

To estimate the financial implications of implementing a guideline in an NH, one must compare the cost of usual care with the cost of care after starting and maintaining the guideline. Researchers have illustrated how the cost of implementing part of the incontinence practice guideline would exceed the cost of usual care in an NH, the latter being ineffective but time-efficient (Schnelle, Keeler, Hays, Simmons, Ouslander, & Siu, 1995).

Based on changing a resident's diapers or clothing one to two times per shift, usual care for an incontinent resident occupies an aide for approximately 7 minutes per shift. Alternatively, prompted voiding can help a resident become more continent, but it requires approximately 22 minutes per shift. The labor costs also include the costs of targeting appropriate residents, training personnel, and managing quality control. Accounting for all costs, an NH would incur an estimated additional $4.30 per resident per day to implement only one aspect of the incontinence guideline (Schnelle et al., 1995). The only financial savings to the NH resulting from this investment would be a slight reduction in laundry costs, which would not offset the costs of following the practice guideline. These labor and cost issues explain why NHs do not consistently sustain guideline-based incontinence programs (Schnelle, McNees, Crooks, & Ouslander, 1995). Such cost barriers could be addressed by reimbursing NHs partly on the basis of the functional outcomes of care. Reductions in incontinence would lead to increased revenue that would offset the NH's costs for following the guideline. The HCFA is currently experimenting with new methods of evaluating the outcomes of NH care, methods that could facilitate outcome-based reimbursement mechanisms in the future (Zimmerman et al., 1995).

Many practice guidelines require that nursing aides and floor nurses consistently carry out new care practices in order to produce and sustain desirable outcomes. For example, the incontinence guideline requires that nursing aides consistently prompt patients about their need for toileting; the pressure sore prevention guideline requires that aides frequently reposition patients. These behaviors can be promoted through an ongoing quality assurance system, featuring

- a monitoring system that accurately and efficiently measures performances
- use of performance data to clearly identify problems, reward success, and suggest improvements
- periodic review of the behaviors to be reinforced

The high turnover of both nursing aides and supervisory nurses requires that training sessions in guideline implementation be frequent and ongoing. The more effective guidelines provide information on how to train providers and use quality assurance techniques to sustain the effects of that training in a highly transient workforce. In addition, the HCFA has recently created an Office of Clinical Standards and Quality, which helps NHs to develop effective quality assurance and improvement projects (see chapter 15). We are optimistic that many of the challenges involved in developing effective internal quality assurance programs for NHs will be resolved.

In summary, practice guidelines offer hope of improving resident outcomes. However, no guideline will improve care unless it addresses the organizational barriers to change discussed throughout this chapter.

Managed Care

Between 1992 and 1997, the number of Medicare enrollees who selected at-risk capitated plans more than tripled from 1.4 million to more than 5 million. Although considerable data support the impression that older persons who enroll in HMOs are healthier than those who remain covered by fee-for-service insurance (Riley, Tudor, Chiang, & Ingber, 1996), some HMO members reside in NHs. Free from the constraints of fee-for-service Medicare reimbursement system, Medicare HMOs can be creative in providing services to their members without fear that such services will be "nonreimbursable." One third of the largest Medicare HMOs have used this opportunity to design innovative programs of comprehensive primary care for their members who reside in NHs.

Virtually all of these programs use nurse practitioners (NPs) or physician assistants (PAs) to augment the care that physicians have traditionally provided in NHs. These HMO programs also typically emphasize the management of acute problems in the NH, whenever possible, and discussions with NH residents and their families about the appropriateness of different levels of intervention (e.g., hospitalization, resuscitation, and palliation). Other features consistent across programs include order-writing capabilities for the NP/PA (which require physicians' countersignatures in some states), the provision of skilled nursing care, health plan approval for physical or occupational therapy, and lack of coverage for transportation to other sites for routine tests or specialty visits. NPs and PAs manage caseloads ranging between 100 and 150 NH residents. These professionals typically participate in the on-call system and are often the first to evaluate residents who have developed acute problems.

Within these broad core elements, plans differ according to three basic models. The first uses a "dedicated team." Its physicians provide only NH, hospice, and home care; none provides hospital or office-based care. The physicians work in pairs with NPs or PAs. The HMO assigns a physician and NP/PA team to each of the nursing homes where HMO members reside. Heikoff (1996) provides a more thorough description of this model.

In the "augmentation" model, physicians provide primary care to NH residents in addition to providing ambulatory and hospital care. NPs augment physicians' capability to provide the NH care. In one example of this model, HMO-employed physicians with large NH practices participate and are released from other clinical responsibilities a half day per month. Usually, each physician follows all of the HMO enrollees who reside at a particular NH. Fama and Fox (1997) provide a more thorough description of this model.

In the "nurse practitioner primary care" model, NPs handle, as care provider and care manager, most day-to-day clinical problems, involving a physician partner as needed or required by state and federal regulations (Fama & Fox, 1997; Malone, Chase, & Bayard, 1993). Usually, NPs are employees of the HMO, whereas physicians receive compensation on a fee-for-service basis.

Researchers have evaluated the effects of these models using historical trends and quasi-experimental designs. Programs that use NPs or PAs appear to provide more primary care visits than do traditional fee-for-service programs. However, not all NP/PA programs have succeeded in reducing hospital or emergency department utilization (Reuben et al., 1998).

In the future, managed care will have increased effects on NHs, and the dynamics that drive managed care will induce change in NH care. In particular, managed care's influence may serve to reduce some of the cost barriers discussed above. Medicare HMOs now reap the benefits of NH practices that result in reduced hospitalizations. If NHs participate in globally capitated integrated networks that include all sites of care, from NHs to acute hospitals, they would probably receive financial incentives to implement practices that reduce costs at other points in the system.

Managed care organizations also have the flexibility to provide NH residents with other services that are not currently reimbursable under fee-for-service rules. Such services will likely have to be of proven benefit in improving patient outcomes before being extended to this population. Although few, if any, interventions fit this description at present, several are in development (e.g., exercise training). Nevertheless, if managed care organizations and NHs were to operate within the same capitated network, they would have considerable incentive to improve NH efficiency without sacrificing quality. Such a stimulus, coupled with dedicated and creative professionals, could result in new and improved models for providing care in NHs.

SUMMARY

Currently, the organization of NHs poses barriers to the appropriate, cost-effective care of NH residents. Evidence-based standards for staff-to-resident ratios do not exist, and a high turnover in the workforce hinders efforts to improve care quality. The relative lack of care expertise among nursing home staff also continues to present a great challenge. Supervising staff members, including floor nurses, directors of nursing, and medical directors, often lack the training, skills, and time needed to promote meaningful change. Organizers of NH care need to search for ways in which to develop a stable, dedicated, and knowledgeable workforce. Few data address the effectiveness of ancillary NH services, such as physical therapy and recreational therapy. Perhaps most significantly, NHs lack financial incentives to invest in programs that improve the quality of care, even if they lead to reduced use of hospitals or other health-related services outside the NH.

Three emerging forces show promise for overcoming these current barriers to effective NH care:

1. *Regulatory efforts.* The MDS and RAP assessment instruments have helped standardize assessment and care planning across NHs. Although these regulatory efforts create paperwork and do not directly address organizational and staffing barriers, some evidence suggests that they improve NH care. Further investigation should address precisely how regulatory efforts bring about organizational change.

2. *Practice guidelines.* Guidelines serve to standardize the care of common conditions afflicting NH residents. For guidelines to work well, they should target only NH residents who are likely to benefit from them. The appropriate situations in which guidelines should be implemented need to be clarified. Unfortunately, the cost to an NH to implement guidelines is often greater than the cost of continuing with usual care. Effective quality assurance programs need to be in place to promote implementation and propagation of guidelines in NH care.

3. *Managed care.* Managed care has the potential to improve NH care through enhanced primary care models and the removal of financial disincentives to innovation. The small number of managed care organizations that have entered into NH care have made extensive use of NPs and PAs, which has increased the amount of primary care that NH residents are receiving. More research should focus on these programs' ability to improve health outcomes and contain costs.

REFERENCES

Abrams, R. C., Teresi, J. A., & Butin, D. N. (1992). Depression in nursing home residents. *Clinics in Geriatric Medicine, 8,* 309–321.

American Association of Retired Persons, Administration on Aging. (1996). *A profile of older Americans: 1996.* Washington, DC: U.S. Department of Health and Human Services.

Bureau of the Census. (1995, May). *Sixty-five plus in the United States* (Statistical Brief No. 94–33). Washington, DC: U.S. Department of Commerce.

Chiodo, L. K., Gerety, M. B., Mulrow, C. D., Rhodes, M. C., & Tuley, M. R. (1992). The impact of physical therapy on nursing home patient outcomes. *Physical Therapy, 72,* 168–175.

Department of Health and Human Services, Public Health Service, National Institutes of Health. (1991, September). *Report to Congress on physical frailty: A reducible barrier to independence for older Americans* (NIH Pub. No. 91-397). Washington, DC: NIH Publications.

Dimant, J. (1991). From quality assurance to quality management in long-term care. *QRB Quality Review Bulletin, 17,* 207–215.

Fama, T., & Fox, P. D. (1997). Efforts to improve primary care delivery to nursing home residents. *Journal of the American Geriatrics Society, 45,* 627–632.

Fries, B. E., Hawes, C., Morris, J. N., Phillips, C., Mor, V., & Park, P. S. (1997). Effect on the national resident assessment instrument on selected health conditions and problems. *Journal of the American Geriatrics Society, 45,* 994–1001.

Heikoff, L. E. (1996). Geriatric care in a large group model. *Current Concepts in Geriatric Managed Care (Kaiser Program) 2,* 4–9.

Institute of Medicine (1986). Improving the Quality of Care in Nursing Homes. National Academy of Science Press Washington, DC.

Kane, R. A., & Kane, R. L. (1987). Long-term care: Principles, programs, and policies. New York: Springer.

Kemper, P., & Murtaugh, C. M. (1991). Lifetime use of nursing home care. *New England Journal of Medicine, 324,* 595–600.

Malone, J. K., Chase, D., & Bayard, J. L. (1993). Caring for nursing home residents. *Journal of Health Care Benefits, 2,* 51–54.

Mercer, S. O., Heacock, P., & Beck, C. (1993). Nurse's aides in nursing homes: Perceptions of training, work loads, racism, and abuse issues. *Journal of Gerontological Social Work, 21,* 95–112.

Molloy, D. W., & Richardson, L. D. (1988). Effects of a three-month exercise program on neuropsychological functioning in elderly institutionalized women: A randomized controlled trial. *Age and Ageing, 17,* 303–310.

Mor, V., Intrator, O., Fries, B. E., Phillips, C., Teno, J., Hiris, J., Hawes, C., & Morris, J. (1997). Changes in hospitalization associated with introducing the resident assessment instrument. *Journal of the American Geriatrics Society, 45,* 1002–1010.

Morris, J. N., Hanes, C., Murphy, K., Nonemaker, S., Phillip, C., Freis, B., & Morris, U. (1991). *Resident assessment instrument, training manual and research guide.* Natick, MA: Eliot Press.

Ouslander, J. G., Schnelle, J. F., Uman, G., Fingold, S., Nigam, J. G., Tuico, E., & Bates-Jensen, B. (1995). Predictors of successful prompted voiding among incontinent nursing home residents. *Journal of the American Medical Association, 273,* 1366–1370.

Panel for Depression Guidelines. (1993). *Depression in primary care: Vol. 2. Treatment of major depression. Clinical practice guideline No. 5* (AHCPR Publication No. 93-0551). Rockville, MD: U.S. Department of Health and Human Services, Agency for Health Care Policy and Research.

Panel for Heart Failure Evaluation and Care of Patients with Left-Ventricular Systolic Dysfunction. (1994). *Heart failure: Evaluation and care of patients with left-ventricular systolic disfunction. Clinical practice guideline No. 11* (AHCPR Publication No. 94-0612). Rockville, MD: U.S. Department of Health and Human Services, Agency for Health Care Policy and Research.

Panel for Prediction and Prevention of Pressure Ulcers in Adults Guidelines.

(1992). *Pressure ulcers in adults: Prediction and prevention. Clinical practice guideline No. 3* (AHCPR Publication 92-0047). Rockville, MD: U.S. Department of Health and Human Services, Agency for Health Care Policy Research.

Panel for Urinary Incontinence in Adult Guidelines. (1996). *Urinary incontinence in adults: Acute and chronic management. Clinical practice guideline No. 2, Update 1996* (AHCPR Publication No. 96-0682). Rockville, MD: U.S. Department of Health and Human Services, Agency for Health Care Policy and Research.

Phillips, C. D., Morris, J. N., Hawes, C., Fries, B. E., Mor, V., Nennstiel, M., & Iannacchione, V. (1997). Association of the Resident Assessment Instrument (RAI) with changes in function, cognition, and psychosocial status. *Journal of the American Geriatrics Society, 45*, 986–993.

Reuben, D. B., Schnelle, J. F., Buchanan, J. L., Kington, R. S., Zellman, G., Farley, D., Hirsch, S. H., Ouslander, J. G. (1997). Primary care of long-stay nursing home residents: Approaches of three health maintenance organizations. Submitted to Journal of the American Geriatrics Society.

Riley, G., Tudor, C., Chiang, Y., & Ingber, M. (1996). Health status of Medicare enrollees in HMOs and fee-for-service in 1994. *Health Care Financial Review, 17*, 67–76.

Rovner, B. W., German, P. S., Brant, L. J., Clark, R., Burton, L., & Folstein, M. F. (1991). Depression and mortality in nursing homes. *Journal of the American Medical Association, 265*, 993–996.

Rovner, B. W., & Katz, I. R. (1994). Neuropsychiatry in nursing homes. In *Textbook of geriatric neuropsychiatry* (pp. 684–693). Cotter, C. E. and Cummings, J. M. (eds) American Psychiatric Press. Washington, DC.

Schnelle, J. F. (1995). Total quality management and the medical director. *Clinics in Geriatric Medicine, 11*, 433–448.

Schnelle, J. F., Cruise, P. A., Rahman, A., & Ouslander, J. G. (1998). Developing rehabilitative behavioral interventions for long-term care: Technology transfer and maintenance issues. *Journal of the American Geriatrics Society.*

Schnelle, J. F., Keeler, E., Hays, R. D., Simmons, S. F., Ouslander, J. G., & Siu, A. L. (1995). A cost utility analysis of two interventions with incontinent nursing home residents. *Journal of the American Geriatrics Society, 43*, 1112–1117.

Schnelle, J. F., MacRae, P. G., Ouslander, J. G., Simmons, S. F., & Nitta, M. A. (1995). Functional incidental training, mobility performance, and incontinence care with nursing home residents. *Journal of the American Geriatrics Society, 43*, 1356–1362.

Schnelle, J. F., McNees, P., Crooks, V., & Ouslander, J. G. (1995). The use of computer-based model to disseminate an incontinence management program. *Gerontologist, 35*, 656–665.

Schnelle, J. F., Ouslander, J. G., & Cruise, P. A. (1997). Policy without technology: A barrier to changing nursing home care. *Gerontologist, 37*, 524–532.

Schnelle, J. F., Ouslander, J. G., & Simmons, S. F. (1993). Predicting nursing home residents' responsiveness to a urinary incontinence treatment protocol. *International Uro-Gynecology Journal, 4*, 89–94.

Schnelle, J. F., Sowell, V. A., Hu, T. W., & Traughber, B. T. (1988). Reduction of urinary incontinence in nursing homes: Does it reduce or increase cost? *Journal of the American Geriatrics Society, 36*, 34–39.

Simmons, S. F., Schnelle, J. F., Uman, G. C., Kulvicki, A. D., Lee, O., & Ouslander, J. G. (1997). Selecting nursing home residents for satisfaction surveys. *Gerontologist, 37,* 543–550.

Strahan, G. W. (1997). *An overview of nursing homes and their current residents: Data from the 1995 National Nursing Home Survey.* (Advance Data from Vital and Health Statistics No. 280). Hyattsville, MD: National Center for Health Statistics.

Tinetti, M. E., Inouye, S. K., Gill, T. M., & Doucette, J. T. (1995). Shared risk factors for falls, incontinence, and functional dependence: Unifying the approach to geriatric syndromes. *Journal of the American Medical Association, 273,* 1348–1353.

Zimmerman, D. R., Karon, S. L., Arling, G., Clark, B. R., Collins, T., Ross, R., & Sainford, F. (1995). The development and testing of nursing home quality indicators. *Health Care Financing Review, 16,* 107–127.

V

Concluding Observations

*T*he changes in American medicine over the past decade have been extraordinary. The pace of change, accelerated by the stillbirth of the Clinton
administration's health plan, could have powerful implications for the care
of older Americans. With encouragement from government, the growth of Medicare
managed care has been extraordinary. Its consequences and its future are discussed
in chapter 18.

One point that will be emphasized is that Medicare HMOs are not homoge-
neous entities. They are a motley array including, among others, traditional
HMOs, loose physician networks, and plans specializing in various aspects of
care like long-term care. Some of the changes associated with Medicare HMOs
could threaten basic American health care values, and the pressures to cut costs
raise concerns about quality. The important issues related to the monitoring of
quality of care and the organized efforts to improve it are discussed in chapter 15.
The pooled capital offers opportunities to invest in new systems of care.

Some tactics used by some managed care organizations (e.g., case managers,
carve-out companies, and disease management programs) could threaten basic
values in American health care, such as the relationship with the personal physician, the integration of services, and the continuity and coordination of care.
These threats are discussed in chapters 16, 17, and 19, along with some creative
efforts by researchers and health plans to use new technologies and care strategies
to meet better the needs of seniors without sacrificing the valued core of medical care.

15

Integrating Quality Assurance Across Sites of Geriatric Care

Eric A. Coleman and Richard W. Besdine

INTRODUCTION

Traditional efforts to ensure quality of health care for older people have been organized according to the location at which care is delivered; integration across sites of care has received minimal attention. Fundamental to ensuring quality is the recognition that over a short period, an older person may receive care at multiple sites from multiple providers for multiple conditions. Movement through different sites of care is synonymous with movement through different—and often isolated—realms of quality standards. While a given care site may warrant some unique approaches to quality assurance, the present fragmented system fails to capture the quality of care experienced by older people. No one has yet refined and implemented information systems that facilitate the transfer of a useful plan of care and the measurement of quality indicators across settings. This fragmentation impedes care coordination and accountability and erodes the trust and confidence of older patients in their caregivers.

This chapter describes several ongoing quality improvement projects, citing existing evidence about whether these efforts result in quality improvement. Although we have organized this discussion by sites of care, we emphasize newer developments designed to foster the organization and integration of quality assessment and improvement across the sites. These newer developments emanate from a broad vision that greater integration of quality assurance is needed to meet the comprehensive acute and long-term care needs of older persons.

QUALITY OF GERIATRIC CARE

Older persons are at risk of receiving care of questionable quality. Recognition that older patients incur high health care costs has stimulated misguided attempts to define quality by utilization reduction rather than by demonstrated improvements in outcomes. Older adults who are burdened by multiple chronic diseases require complex care. In addition, challenges to accessing care, including communicative barriers (vision and hearing), cognitive impairment, mobility impairment, and inadequate transportation, are common. These challenges are greater for ethnically diverse or financially disadvantaged older populations. Few delivery systems have much experience in caring for frail older adults (Epstein, 1995). Although more fully integrated delivery systems offer the potential for improving the coordination of health care services, a well-organized, comprehensive system for caring for older persons does not yet exist (Kramer, Fox, & Morgenstern, 1992; Wagner, 1996).

Much of the recent attention to quality of geriatric care has focused on highly publicized comparisons of health outcomes between payment systems (i.e., managed care vs. fee-for-service) (Carlisle et al., 1992; Clement, Retchin, Brown, & Stegall, 1994; Shaughnessesy, Schlenker, & Hitke, 1994; Ware, Bayliss, Rogers, Kosinski, & Tarlov, 1996). While these studies may provide insight into how payment structure influences the provision of care, any significant average differences in measurable quality are small in comparison to the wide variation in quality within payment systems. Neither payment system provides a model for high-quality geriatric care; attention to differences between them detracts from their common need for substantial improvement in outcomes.

MEDICARE: QUALITY ASSURANCE EFFORTS

As the largest purchaser of health care services for older adults (nearly $200 billion in 1996), the Medicare program must play a central role in ensuring quality of care. The Health Care Financing Administration (HCFA) underwent dramatic restructuring in the first half of 1997, including creation of a new component—the Office of Clinical Standards and Quality. The central theme of the reorganization is to structure all activities, including quality assessment and improvement, according to beneficiaries' needs, rather than provider type or locus of care.

HCFA's Quality Improvement Program aspires to measure quality based on performance. After setting beneficiary-centered priorities in health care, HCFA collects and analyzes baseline data about performance to identify opportunities to improve care. To actually improve care, HCFA can intervene by (1) establishing and enforcing performance standards (setting the minimum threshold that care purchased by HCFA must surpass), (2) providing technical assistance for improvement to plans and providers (largely through the network of Quality Improvement Organizations [QIOs], previously known as Peer Review Organizations [PROs]), (3) giving consumers information about quality that they value and can use to make choices, (4) making quality-oriented payment and coverage decisions, and (5) rewarding desired performance. The Quality Improvement Program is dynamic, fed by information from the analysis of performance data; continual reevaluation and revision of priorities for quality improvement will be most responsive to the needs of Medicare beneficiaries.

Medicare is moving toward measuring quality across care settings (e.g., hospitals and nursing homes), allowing comparisons to benchmarks, identification of opportunities to improve care, and wide replication of successful interventions. The main goal is to establish a common set of indicators that can measure performance across sites—hospital, nursing home, post-acute care, rehabilitation, and home care. This information will then be made available to HCFA central and regional offices, states, QIOs, providers, and purchasers. Beneficiaries and their advocates should find the information useful in making informed provider choices (see also chapter 19).

HCFA has traditionally maintained quality assurance activities through reliance on external strategies, setting a minimum "floor" for quality and upholding these standards through inspection and enforcement. More recently, HCFA has begun to emphasize internal quality assurance strategies that encourage plans and provider organizations to generate their own internal quality improvement projects. All Conditions of Participation in Medicare (regulations that define the responsibilities of organizations that provide care to Medicare beneficiaries, applying to both managed care and fee-for-service arrangements) will now require quality assurance using a system of Quality Assessment and Performance Improvement (QAPI). By design, QAPI encourages plans and providers of care to identify opportunities to improve care, measure baseline performance in a given area of quality, design and implement a plan for improvement, and remeasure to determine whether improvement has occurred. This approach combines HCFA's goal of increasing performance-based quality improvement efforts with the principles of continuous quality improvement, whereby providers and plans seek quality improvements in outcomes most critical to the health status of their particular populations.

The End Stage Renal Disease (ESRD) Program illustrates HCFA's multifaceted approach to quality assurance and improvement. HCFA promulgates and publishes minimum standards, conditions of participation in ESRD, for all organizations providing services to its beneficiaries.

In addition to setting minimum performance standards, the newest version for each provider type specifies a QAPI algorithm as well. The regional networks funded in the program provide technical assistance in quality improvement projects for ESRD. Consumers receive information through a "Know Your Number" initiative that encourages ESRD beneficiaries to track their urea removal rate (a measure of the effectiveness of each dialysis episode) and advocate for themselves when values are low. Currently in progress is a payment demonstration that capitates dialysis services and allows providers to share in savings resulting from better dialysis and concomitant lower hospitalization rates. Finally, a newly developed initiative designates high-performing dialysis centers as "facilities of achievement," a reward for good performance.

INPATIENT QUALITY ASSURANCE

Efforts to improve the quality of inpatient hospital care for older adults have largely inhabited the domain of the QIOs. The QIOs have evolved toward a more collaborative relationship with hospitals and providers, bringing evidence-based care strategies and evaluative research into the mainstream of care. Currently, 53 QIOs nationwide are conducting more than 250 active quality improvement projects. The prototype of the QIO initiatives has been the Health Care Quality Improvement Program (HCQIP) (Jencks & Wilensky, 1992). As an evolving strategy aimed at quality improvement, HCQIP has collaborated with clinicians and professional societies to identify strategies for implementing interventions that will improve outcomes of care for common and important conditions afflicting Medicare beneficiaries.

Evidence that HCQIP is an effective means for improving quality of care is expanding. The most elaborate of the projects has been the Cooperative Cardiovascular Project (CCP) (Ellerbeck et al., 1995), which began as a pilot in four states and now is being widely replicated. The CCP's main goal is to demonstrate an increase in the use of beta blockers and aspirin following hospitalization for myocardial infarction. The data analyzed thus far look very promising (Health Care Financing Administration, 1997). Collaborative efforts between the QIO and the health care community in Oregon led to a near 50% reduction in medication errors among older patients (Vladeck, 1994). A QIO project in the State of New York demonstrated a reduction in rates of unnecessary right heart catheterization and a commensurate drop in complication rates (Malach & Nenner, 1996). The lessons learned from HCQIP will be valuable for improving quality not only in hospitals but also in other sites of care. The adaptation of the HCQIP approach to nonhospital sites of care will greatly advance a more uniform strategy for quality assurance.

AMBULATORY QUALITY ASSURANCE

Although historically quality assurance has emphasized inpatient care, recent efforts have begun to include ambulatory care in performance measurement and quality improvement. Weiner and associates stimulated greater attention to ambulatory care after analyzing Medicare claims and demonstrating that office-based quality for Medicare beneficiaries with diabetes was disappointingly low (Weiner et al., 1995). In response, the Medicare Managed Care Quality Improvement Program (MMCQIP) has initiated a quality improvement strategy for outpatient diabetes care, using performance measures of retinal screening exams and foot evaluations, to detect early signs of complications.

The National Committee on Quality Assurance (NCQA) has collaborated with the HCFA to ensure that the Health Plan Employer Data Information System (HEDIS) includes performance measures that are directly relevant to the ambulatory care of Medicare beneficiaries in managed care plans (National Committee on Quality Assurance, 1996). The HCFA now requires participating health plans to collect, report, and be accountable for data reflecting the ambulatory care received by older adults (e.g., longitudinal assessment of functional status, breast cancer screening, retinal exams for diabetics, flu shots, advice to quit smoking, beta-blocker use after myocardial infarction, and ambulatory follow-up after hospitalization for mental illness) (see also chapter 3).

Formed in 1995 by large public and private purchasers of health care to endorse performance measures, the Foundation for Accountability (FAcct) is leading another effort to develop measures of quality that address the unique care needs of older adults. Like HEDIS, FAcct strives to guide consumers and purchasers in making informed selections among providers. However, rather than encompassing a broad set of diseases and procedures, the FAcct measures will emphasize the importance of functional status in guiding treatment decisions and care coordination across the different sites of care. While HEDIS performance measures are specific to the delivery of managed care, FAcct designed its performance measures to apply to the delivery of fee-for-service care as well, with accompanying accountability.

QUALITY ASSURANCE IN NURSING HOMES

The single most influential event in raising the quality of care in nursing homes has been the implementation of the Omnibus Budget Reconciliation Act of 1987 (OBRA '87). As a result of OBRA '87, the focus of quality assurance in nursing homes has shifted from structural requirements for the facility and staff ratios for the providers to the resident's quality of life and the outcomes of the care provided (Zimmerman et al., 1995). Although full implementation did not begin until July 1995, accumulating evidence suggests that OBRA '87 has positively affected the care received by older nursing home residents. Physical restraint of nursing home residents has declined by nearly 50% (Gagel, 1995). Inappropriate use of antipsychotic medications has decreased by 25% to 36% (Garrard, Chen, & Dowd, 1995; Rovner, Edelman, Cox, & Shmuely, 1992; Schorr, Fought, & Ray, 1994). Studies have documented a 50% reduction in dehydration, a 30% decrease in the use of indwelling urinary catheters, and a 25% decline in hospitalization rates among nursing home residents (Vladeck, 1996). Although the first round of inspections found that 70% of facilities were out of compliance with OBRA '87, 80% avoided penalties by implementing adequate plans of correction.

As a direct result of OBRA '87, the HCFA required a standardized assessment of physical and functional status—the Minimum Data Set (MDS)—for all residents (see also chapter 17). The MDS assessment generates patient-centered quality indicators (e.g., recovery of physical function after fracture, and management of depression, and management of incontinence) that guide quality improvement efforts. Applying these indicators to all residents in all facilities (with adequate risk adjustment) enables the HCFA to provide each nursing home with data about its performance in relation to national standards and to compare state and national averages. Purchasers, consumers, and consumer advocates also will be extremely interested in these performance data.

The quality improvement activities of the QIOs will soon expand into the nursing home setting. Similar to the approach used in hospital settings, nursing homes will develop their own internal quality assessment and improvement activities in collaboration with the QIOs, using performance measures derived from the MDS. This internal focus will permit providers to identify quality improvement projects directed toward the facility's unique population (e.g., residents with Alzheimer's disease, stroke, or urinary incontinence) and the facility's most pressing problems.

Using performance measurement to guide and evaluate quality improvement has the potential to improve care across all sites in which beneficiaries receive service. Similar approaches to quality improvement in different settings of care allow the linking of data on performance measures across sites. For example, the Uniform Needs Assessment Instrument (UNAI), which is completed at the time of hospital discharge, contains many of the same core quality indicators as the nursing home MDS. Efforts are also under way to standardize elements of measurement for home health care.

QUALITY ASSURANCE IN HOME HEALTH CARE

In the 1990s, home health care has exploded to a $20 billion per year industry, yet we know little about its effectiveness (see also chapters 5 and

12). Older adults generally express strong preferences for receiving care in their homes rather than in institutions. Unique aspects in the delivery of home care have implications for quality assessment and accountability. Older patients exert more control over their medical and nursing regimens in the home, and their level of participation and adherence to the plan of care influences performance results positively or negatively. Often services received are a combination of formal and informal care from skilled and unskilled health care workers, family members, and friends. Defining what constitutes a discrete episode of home care is challenging, as the older person may be hospitalized after home care has begun. Determining the extent to which the home health agency is accountable for particular outcomes of care requires adjustment for these differences.

A recent survey of Medicare claims data examined patterns of home health care use. It found no support for the claim that services provided in the home replace hospital services; instead, services appeared to provide long-term care. The authors concluded that the wide geographic variation in home health care use suggests a lack of consensus about its appropriate use (Welch, Wennberg, & Welch, 1996). Evaluation of Medicare-reimbursed episodes of home care found substantial quality deficiencies and actual or potential adverse consequences (Jette, Smith, & McDermott 1996). The complexity of patients' care needs correlated strongly with the likelihood and severity of quality problems.

Recent developments in home health care will likely enhance the evidence base for measuring its effectiveness. HCFA will require all home health agencies to perform patient assessments that incorporate the Outcomes Assessment Information Set (OASIS) on all clients. OASIS is not a comprehensive assessment instrument, but rather a core set of measures from which quality indicators can be derived. Indicators in development will reflect more relevant outcomes of home health care, such as the percent of patients who improve in ambulation following surgery for hip fracture. The researchers who developed OASIS have demonstrated the value of uniform performance measurement in comparing home health care outcomes (Shaughnessey et al., 1994). Using risk adjustment to compare fee-for-service and managed care home health agencies, they found a direct association among the intensity of services received, associated costs, and improved clinical outcomes of care.

QUALITY ASSURANCE IN POSTACUTE CARE

Built around reducing inpatient stays, postacute care continues to proliferate nationally as a profitable industry (see also chapter 8). While definitions of postacute care abound, most encompass the concept of goal-oriented interdisciplinary services provided in place of all or part of an acute hospitalization (Harvell, 1996). Quality assurance efforts within postacute care have staggered, however, due to uncertainty concerning (1) a uniform definition of postacute care, (2) which patients' needs are best met in this level of care, and (3) how postacute care differs from other types of care. As a result, measurable outcomes of care still lack definition and uniform measurement instruments. To date, no rigorous study has documented improved outcomes of transfer to postacute care when compared to alternatives (e.g., an additional 1 to 2 days in the hospital or transfer to traditional nursing home or home care). Kramer and colleagues (1997) compared functional outcomes of care for older adults with stroke and hip fracture depending on whether they were discharged to a rehabilitation facility, a subacute unit in skilled nursing facility, or a traditional nursing home. Whereas patients with stroke experienced better functional outcomes at 6 months when discharged to rehabilitation facilities, the functional outcomes of patients with hip fractures did not vary significantly among the respective three sites (see also chapter 9).

The Joint Commission on Accreditation of Health Care Organizations (JCAHO) has developed accreditation standards for postacute care modeled on nursing home standards. Several trade organizations have drafted clinical standards as guidelines for the organization and delivery of services and for outcomes measures (Harvell, 1996). Comparisons across different structural arrangements require well-defined measurable quality outcomes for postacute care. Since Medicare is by far the largest purchaser of postacute care, performance measurement probably will become the driving force for quality assurance, as part of the HCFA's integrated strategy for quality improvement.

PRIVATE SECTOR QUALITY ASSURANCE

In the preceding sections, we have emphasized the HCFA's role in ensuring quality in health care for older adults, either through external regulatory approaches or through encouraging provider organizations to develop their own internal quality assurance initiatives. Organizations have arisen where external quality improvement efforts leave off—supporting providers and plans in developing their own internal quality initiatives. The Institute for Healthcare Improvement (IHI) is an independent, nonprofit organization that emphasizes collaboration rather than competition among provider organizations in advancing quality improvement (Berwick, 1996). The IHI motivates provider organizations and plans to develop its own internal CQI programs in concert with the HCFA. One example of the IHI's efforts particularly relevant to older adults is a 40-hospital collaborative project to reduce adverse drug events (Borzo, 1997; Institute for

Healthcare Improvement, 1997). Through efforts that focus on improving the design and function of systems to better support achieving desirable outcomes of care, this project demonstrated an 85% reduction in medication transcription and prescribing errors.

OLDER CONSUMERS AND QUALITY OF CARE

The expectation that a more informed public will demand a higher quality of care has fueled a growing recognition of the older consumer's role in quality assurance. Accordingly, performance measures need to incorporate values commonly held by older adults (e.g., maintenance of independence). Furthermore, it is essential that older consumers find these measures understandable and compelling; health plans' use of the information (i.e., in marketing) also needs adequate oversight. While evidence for a direct correlation between quality and satisfaction does not yet exist, focus groups of Medicare beneficiaries reveal that older consumers often define quality of care in terms of satisfaction and the quality of interpersonal care and communication that they receive from their providers (Lohr, Donaldson, & Walker, 1991). Outcome measurement strategies should incorporate these domains. Efforts aimed at educating older adults so that they can become more participatory health consumers will become increasingly important.

CONCLUSIONS

The assurance of quality care for older adults as they move across sites of care delivery requires comprehensive standardized patient assessment, in conjunction with performance measurement of the care provided. Currently, efforts are under way to develop and implement the information systems needed to track older persons as they move through the delivery system and to link the relevant data and patient preferences across all providers of care. Performance measurement then can follow, promoting the delivery of high-quality care and accountability. More than ever before, health services research that focuses on changes in health outcomes as older adults make transitions between types and locations of care will benefit both older persons and society (Institute of Medicine, 1996).

ACKNOWLEDGEMENT

The authors would like to recognize the invaluable advice of Stephen F. Jencks, M.D., and Thomas Marciniak of the Office of Clinical Standards and Quality, Health Care Financing Administration, in the preparation of this chapter.

REFERENCES

Berwick, D. M. (1996). Quality comes home. *Annals of Internal Medicine, 125,* 839–843.

Borzo, G. (1997, April 21). Pink slip for prescriptions. *American Medical News,* pp. 3, 31.

Carlisle, D. M., Siu, A. L., Keeler, E. B., McGlynn, E. A., Rubenstein, L. Z., & Brook, R. H. (1992). HMO vs. fee-for-service care for older persons with myocardial infarction. *American Journal of Public Health, 82,* 1626–1630.

Clement, D. G., Retchin, S. M., Brown, R. S., & Stegall, M. H. (1994). Access and outcomes of elderly patients enrolled in managed care. *Journal of the American Medical Association, 271,* 1487–1492.

Ellerbeck, E. F., Jencks, S. F., Radford, M. J., Kresowik, T. F., Craig, A. S., Gold, J. A., Krumholz H. M., & Vogel, R. A. (1995). Quality of care for Medicare patients with acute myocardial infarction. *Journal of the American Medical Association, 273,* 1509–1514.

Epstein, A. (1995). Performance reports on quality—prototypes, problems and QI aspects. *New England Journal of Medicine, 333,* 57–61.

Gagel, B. J. (1995). Health Care Quality Improvement Program: A new approach. *Health Care Financing Review, 16,* 15–23.

Garrard, J., Chen, V., & Dowd, B. (1995). The impact of the 1987 federal regulations on the use of psychotropic drugs in Minnesota nursing homes. *American Journal of Public Health, 85,* 771–776.

Harvell, J. (1996). Subacute care: Its role and the assurance of quality. In R. J. Newcomer & A. M. Wilkinson (Eds.). *Annual review of gerontology and geriatrics: Focus on managed care and quality assurance* (pp. 37–59). New York: Springer.

Institute for Healthcare Improvement. (1997). *Reducing adverse drug events.* St. Louis: National Congress.

Institute of Medicine. Feasley, J. C. (Ed.). (1996). *Health outcomes for older people: Questions for the coming decade.* Washington, DC: National Academy Press.

Jencks, S. F., & Wilensky, G. R. (1992). The health care quality improvement initiative: A new approach to quality assurance in Medicare. *Journal of the American Medical Association, 268,* 900–903.

Jette, A. M., Smith, K. W., & McDermott, S. M. (1996). Quality of Medicare-reimbursed home care. *Gerontologist, 36,* 492–501.

Kramer, A. M., Fox, P. D., & Morgenstern, N. (1992). Geriatric care approaches in health maintenance organizations. *Journal of the American Geriatrics Society, 40,* 1055–1067.

Kramer, A. M., Steiner, J. F., Schlenker, R. E., Eilertsen, T. B., Hrincevich, C. A., Tropea D. A., Ahmad, L. A., & Eckhoff, D. G. (1997). Outcomes and costs after hip fracture and stroke: A comparison of rehabilitation settings. *Journal of the American Medical Association, 277,* 396–404.

Lohr, K. N., Donaldson, M. S., & Walker, A. J. (1991). Medicare: A strategy for quality assurance: beneficiary and physician focus groups. *Quality Review Bulletin, 8,* 242–253.

Malach, M., Nenner R. P. & Paschal, J. I. (1998). Impact of an Educational Program on Bilateral Heart Catherization Patterns. *American Journal of Medical Quality* (in Press).

Marciniak, T. A., Ellerbeeck, E. F., Radford, M. J., Kresowik, T. F., Gold, J. A., Krumholz, H. M., Kiefec, C. L., Allman, R. M., Vogel, R. A., and Jencks, S. F. (1998). Improving the quality of care for Medicare patients with acute myocardial infarction. *Journal of the American Medical Association* (in Press).

National Committee for Quality Assurance (1997). Health Plan Employer Data and Information Set (HEDIS), version 3.0/1998 Washington D.C.

Rovner, B. W., Edelman, B. A., Cox, M. P., & Shmuely, Y. (1992). The impact of antipsychotic drug regulations on psychotropic prescribing practices in nursing homes. *American Journal of Psychiatry, 149,* 1390–1392.

Schorr, R. I., Fought, R. L., & Ray, W. A. (1994). Changes in antipsychotic drug use in nursing homes during implementation of the OBRA-87 regulations. *Journal of the American Medical Association, 271,* 358–362.

Shaughnessey, P. W., Schlenker, R. E., & Hitke, D. A. (1994). Home health care outcomes under capitated and fee-for-service payment. *Health Care Financing Review, 16,* 187–221.

Vladeck, B. C. (1994). The health care quality improvement program: A progress report. *Journal of the American Medical Association, 271,* 1896.

Vladeck, B. C. (1996). The past, present and future of nursing home quality. *Journal of the American Medical Association, 275,* 425.

Wagner, E. H. (1996). The promise and performance of HMOs in improving outcomes in older adults. *Journal of the American Geriatrics Society, 44,* 1251–1257.

Ware, J. E., Bayliss, M. S., Rogers, W. H., Kosinski, M., & Tarlov A. R. (1996). Differences in 4-year health outcomes for elderly and poor, chronically ill patients treated in HMO and fee-for-service systems. *Journal of the American Medical Association, 276,* 1039–1047.

Weiner, J. P., Parente, S. T., Garnick, D. W., Fowles, J., Lawthers A. G., & Palmer, R. H. (1995). Variation in office-based quality: A claims profile of care provided to Medicare patients with diabetes. *Journal of the American Medical Association, 273,* 1503–1508.

Welch, H. G., Wennberg, D. E., & Welch, W. P. (1996). The use of Medicare home health care services. *New England Journal of Medicine, 335,* 324–329.

Zimmerman, D. R., Karon, S. L., Arling, G., Clark, B. R., Collins T., Ross, R., & Sainfort, F. (1995). Development and testing of nursing quality indicators. *Health Care Financing Review, 16,* 107–127.

16

Integrating Care

Chad Boult and James T. Pacala

> The true test of these efforts is whether the care of patients is optimized
> as a consequence. It is far more difficult to develop a delivery system
> that provides high-quality, thoroughly coordinated, and cost-effective
> care than it is to acquire facilities, create governing bodies, and
> decide who will be the institution's chief executive officer.
> —(Kassirer, 1996, pp. 722–723)

It is one thing to assert that older people, especially those with complex
conditions, need comprehensive health care that spans several sites, professions, organizations, and funding mechanisms. It is quite another to
deliver such care in a coordinated, efficient manner. Despite the best of
intentions, the addition of more care often increases communication errors,
duplication of effort, administrative burden, financial challenge, and even
adverse outcomes. The fragmentation of health care for chronically ill
seniors in the traditional fee-for-service system is notorious. Thus, in creating new systems of comprehensive care, the builders need to attend
seriously to integration, lest their efforts only recreate novel—and potentially more expensive—versions of today's chaos.

INTEGRATION OF PRIMARY CARE

On the front lines, physicians have traditionally focused on medical conditions, nurses on education, and social workers on counseling and
arranging community services. Rarely have these or other health professionals communicated effectively with one another, let alone integrated
their plans and services for patients with complex needs. However, psychosocial, educational, and other nonmedical factors influence, at least as
powerfully as physicians' care, these seniors' health status and their need

for expensive health-related services. Simultaneously, the array of interventions designed to address these challenges must be coordinated in order to be maximally effective and efficient.

One approach to coordinating complex primary care is to entrust it to teams. At the core of the typical team are a physician, a nurse, and a social worker, or alternate professionals with equivalent skills. Depending on patients' needs, a team may also include dietitians, pharmacists, psychologists, health educators, case managers, physical therapists, occupational therapists, and dentists. In some cases, the patients' family members or friends who provide "informal" care play important roles.

Group discussion provides a vehicle for integrating team members' evaluations, recommendations, and actions. The individual members have their own discrete domains of expertise and responsibility, and they share parts of domains with other members (e.g., physicians and pharmacists both address medications; nurses, social workers, and informal caregivers address functional limitations). Leadership designation varies by team and by the patient being treated. On some teams, the physician is the leader; on others, a consultant. Ideally, the various professionals' leadership roles change according to the needs of individual patients. For a patient with predominantly medical needs, the physician would logically lead the team and assume primary responsibility for integrating the efforts of the other team members. Alternately, if social or educational needs were primary, the social worker or nurse would assume the leadership role.

Researchers have tested the team approach within many types of care settings. Table 16.1 lists the most recent studies. Because of operational or financial constraints, some care systems have difficulty bringing all team members together for meetings. As an alternative, some are experimenting with a model in which a single team member with geriatrics expertise integrates the team's efforts. As chapter 4 describes in greater detail, teams of the future, more consistently than those of years past, will rely on evidence-based goals, priorities, instruments, and treatment methods.

Although teams bring considerable expertise to the care of seniors with complex needs, they also bring challenges. A team's creation and operation require time, training, resources, and the revision of traditional roles. Professionals from different disciplines must learn each other's languages, values, background, skills, and work habits. They must learn to respect, appreciate, and rely on each other. Attainment of effective team functioning requires that our systems of medical education and health care delivery commit resources to the training and maintenance of teams. The ultimate success or failure of a geriatric team will probably derive from the skills of its individual members, their ability to coordinate their efforts, and their efficiency in applying their expertise to those seniors whose needs are complex enough to warrant such a significant investment of resources.

TABLE 16.1   Studies of the Team Approach

Type of Care Environment	Authors	Year(s)
Primary care	Beck et al.	1997
	Eng et al.	1997
Home care	Melin et al.	1993
Comprehensive geriatric assessment (CGA)	Reuben et al.	1995
Geriatric evaluation and management (GEM)	Boult et al.	1998
Case management	Rich et al.	1995
Acute hospital care	Landefeld	1995
Subacute care	vonSternberg et al.	1997
Long-term care	Fama & Fox	1997

INTEGRATION OF SPECIALIST CARE

At times, the expertise of specialist physicians may improve the outcomes experienced by seniors with serious, complicated, or unusual conditions. At other times, chronically ill seniors and their families may find the care provided by multiple specialists (including geriatricians) or special programs to be fragmented, duplicative, confusing, and logistically stressful. Chapters 3 and 4 review the debate about the optimal role of specialty care for complex patients. For which patients should specialists provide primary care, and for which should they provide consultation? How many specialists or specialized programs can serve a patient before the benefit of their collective expertise dwindles beneath the complexity and costs of receiving care from multiple sources? How should CGA programs integrate with primary care services? No one knows the ideal approach to integrating specialist and generalist care, but new models should strive for

- patient-centeredness, in which care systems organize around the needs of patients instead of vice versa, and
- alignment of incentives, under which specialists and generalists all receive fair rewards for good patient outcomes.

The latter principle would also encourage increased collegiality, respect, cooperation, and learning between specialist and generalist physicians.

INTEGRATION OF COMMUNITY-BASED AND HEALTH SYSTEM–BASED CARE

Much of the care that affects the well-being of frail older persons comes not from health professionals at all, but from publicly supported nonprofit agencies: senior centers, religious and civic organizations, diagnosis-related support groups (e.g., the Alzheimer's Association), day care centers, Meals-on-Wheels programs, congregate dining, home modification programs, transportation services, chore services, companion services, and financial services. City, county, and state health departments often provide home care, case management, adult protection, and other services. The integration of these public resources with those provided by commercial health care systems seems crucial, but it represents another set of logistical and financial challenges. How should case managers, nurses, and social workers employed by health care organizations interact with those employed by local agencies or health departments in arranging and coordinating clients' services? How many such providers should a person have, and who should pay for them? While some community-based organizations have developed mutually satisfactory collaborative relationships with managed care organizations, others are concerned that HMOs and provider organizations are attempting to use more publicly supported services than community budgets can afford. In the future, community and commercial organizations together must find new and creative models for developing, providing, and coordinating optimal combinations of services and for sharing their costs equitably.

INTEGRATION ACROSS SITES OF CARE

The assurance of continuity across diverse sites of care is inherent to integrating the efforts of multiple practitioners and organizations. Hospitals, nursing homes, emergency rooms, ambulatory offices, pharmacies, home care agencies, outpatient surgery and rehabilitation centers, laboratories, transportation services, and vendors of medical equipment all provide care, but often they do not interact effectively with each other. Each may offer patients different sets of goals, plans, and providers of care. Clinical and financial information is gathered separately by individual providers, recorded in widely varying formats, transferred unreliably, duplicated repeatedly, and lost frequently—even among providers within the same organization.

The primacy of some providers' alignments with specific insurance companies, regulatory agencies, and with other providers—more than with patients' needs—only perpetuates the disjointed nature of this "nonsystem" of care. Future steps toward resolution of such disintegration should

- commit to the view that the patient is the customer
- develop interdisciplinary teams within which one provider assumes responsibility for ensuring that each patient's care is appropriate and accessible

- create financial and regulatory incentives that encourage cooperation among health care providers
- develop standardized electronic databases that are appropriately
  secure yet accessible to providers
- adopt evidence-based, transfacility, clinical pathways

INTEGRATION OF FINANCING

One of the most powerful and pervasive disincentives to clinical integration is the multiplicity of mechanisms for financing health care. Frequently,
a chronically ill older person obtains services through a combination of
personal savings, commercial insurance, and programs supported by federal, state, and local funds. Typically, each party attempts to preserve its
resources as much as possible, shifting costs to the others whenever it
can. Patients are often caught in the middle, bewildered by a morass of
legalistic rules and red tape. The confusion may deny them services from
which they could benefit and to which they are actually entitled. Similarly,
providers of care are frustrated by a myriad of ever-changing insurance
coverages, reimbursement rates, and billing requirements imposed by
the many third parties with whom they must negotiate in order to retain
their patients.

MODELS OF INTEGRATED CARE

Growing interest and sizable investment is fueling ongoing experiments
designed to achieve better integration of health services, especially for
persons with complex needs. Progress is slow and difficult, however,
because the required changes are daunting, and we have few hard outcome data to guide us. Eventual integration will probably require that our
present finance-oriented systems of care (see Figure 16.1) evolve into new
client-oriented systems (see Figure 16.2).

In today's finance-centered system, specific funds (e.g., Medicare Part
A) support specific programs (e.g., postacute care) that provide specific
services (e.g,. physical therapy) to specific subgroups (Medicare beneficiaries who have just spent 3 or more days in a hospital). When the needs
for care arise, clients (or their families) must quickly learn which services
are recommended and available, who could provide them, which (if any)
fund will pay for them, and how to arrange them, complete the paperwork, and coordinate them with other needed services. Well-educated,
assertive, healthy people with only occasional needs for care often obtain
good service, but chronically ill people with multiple ongoing needs and

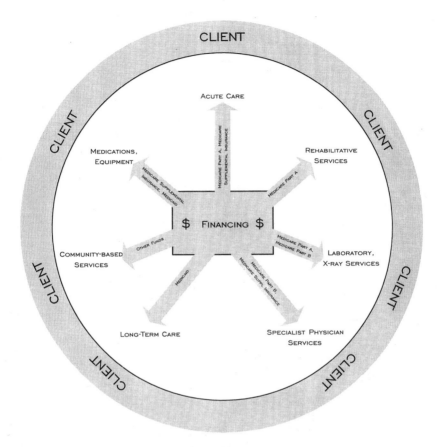

FIGURE 16.1 "Finance-oriented" system of care. Client must logistically circumnavigate a financially centered dispersion of payers and services to piece together his or her own health care.

little understanding of how to make the system work for them are often overwhelmed and underserved.

A client-oriented system (see Figure 16.2) would simplify the client's role; a client would consider the options presented by a primary provider or case manager, select some, and then focus on using them to recover health and functional ability. The case manager or primary provider would integrate (through information systems, practice guidelines, and collaborative professional relationships) and coordinate the services that the client selected.

First steps toward integrated health care for seniors are now occurring as HMOs assume the risk of paying for all of the acute care for increasing numbers of Medicare beneficiaries in return for capitated payments from the U.S. Health Care Financing Administration (HCFA). More than 15% of

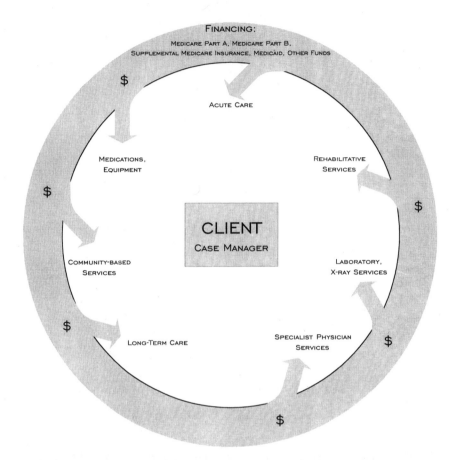

FIGURE 16.2 **"Client-oriented" system of care. Through the case manager, client obtains a set of coordinated services financed by pooled monies.**

all Medicare beneficiaries are now enrolled in such Medicare HMOs, and total enrollment is growing at about 100,000 persons per month. The responsibility for the costs of the health care of older people with complex needs—and the competitive pressures of the marketplace—have given the participating HMOs strong incentives to integrate the efforts of those who provide that health care. In response, most large Medicare HMOs have begun case management programs (see chapter 4), and some have also begun to improve their capacity to provide medical care that is integrated across various delivery sites. The most progressive organizations are developing information systems, clinical guidelines, interdisciplinary teams, and contractual arrangements to facilitate the continuity of care across outpatient offices, subacute care units, emergency rooms, acute care hospitals, rehabilitation programs, home care services, and nursing homes.

EXAMPLES OF SYSTEMS THAT INTEGRATE ACUTE AND LONG-TERM CARE

As long as HCFA continues to offer attractive capitation incentives, capitated health care organizations will continue attempting to integrate their systems for delivering acute care to older persons. The integration of acute and long-term services, however, will require even more profound changes. Realizing that "form follows funding," HCFA has spawned at least three ambitious experiments designed to stimulate such comprehensive integration. Each project relies on pooled, capitated dollars that traditional fee-for-service Medicare and Medicaid programs expend separately to purchase circumscribed sets of services for older people who have become ill. HCFA policymakers and administrators hope that the approach will reduce incentives to shift costs and increase provider organizations' flexibility to develop creative, proactive systems for delivering effective, integrated comprehensive acute and long-term care.

PACE: The Program of All-Inclusive Care of the Elderly

In the first of these experiments, HCFA approved capitated Medicare and Medicaid payments to On Lok Inc., an organization that agreed to provide all acute and long-term care for several hundred seniors (55 years or older) in San Francisco who were eligible for nursing home care (Eng, Pedulla, Eleazer, McCann, & Fox, 1997). On Lok's integrated system, coordinated through an adult day health center, provides primary care by an interdisciplinary team; specialty care by contract; and, when necessary, home care, medications, diagnostic testing, transportation, durable medical equipment, chore services, and care in hospitals and nursing homes. Early reports of On Lok's ability to provide cost-effective comprehensive health care has led to its replication at 19 demonstration sites during the first half of the 1990s. Now known as the Program of All-Inclusive Care of the Elderly, or PACE, this program is being replicated in dozens of cities around the United States.

The 2,700 frail seniors who are now enrolled in PACE are, on average, 80 years old with 7 to 8 medical conditions and 2.7 ADL limitations; 42% are demented. They agree to receive all of their health care from (or by referral from) a PACE interdisciplinary team comprising an internist or family physician, a nurse practitioner, nurses, social workers, recreation therapists, a physical therapist, an occupational therapist, and a dietitian. They also agree to use, if needed, one hospital, one nursing home, one pharmacy, and one panel of specialists with whom PACE has contractual relationships.

New enrollees undergo an initial comprehensive assessment; thereafter, with the help of the PACE transportation system, they attend the PACE adult day health care center 2 or 3 days each week. There, they socialize, eat lunch, are monitored for physical, functional, and emotional decline, and receive treatment as needed from appropriate members of the team. They see their PACE physician monthly, get reassessed by their team quarterly, and when necessary, receive care at home, in the hospital, or in the nursing home. Their providers encourage them to complete advance directives.

Capitated payments from HCFA and state Medicaid funds cover most of the costs of the PACE services. The HCFA payments are set at Medicare's average adjusted per capita cost (AAPCC), multiplied by a factor of 2.39; the Medicaid payments are negotiated state by state. The combined revenue, which averaged $3,388 per member per month in 1994, must cover the costs of the large interdisciplinary team and the adult day health care center, as well as those of all of the services listed above. Nevertheless, because of low hospital and nursing home utilization rates, total revenues exceeded total costs at most PACE sites. A cost-effectiveness study is under way, but its findings are not yet available. In a recent study of the quality of care provided at eight PACE sites, practicing geriatricians and GNPs performed extensive reviews of PACE charts. The reviewers judged overall quality of care to be equal to or better than community standards in 92% of cases. After 6 to 12 months of PACE care, most (79%) of the PACE patients fared as well as or better than predicted on the basis of their clinical condition at baseline. However, the quality of care varied significantly across the eight sites, three of the sites showing consistently poorer ratings than the other five (Pacala, Kane, Smith, & Atherly, 1998).

The PACE experiment is a creative attempt to overcome several formidable obstacles to providing cost-effective complex health care. By accepting federal and state capitation payments and the full financial risk of providing all acute and long-term health care needed by their enrollees, the PACE sites have strong incentives to avert the need for expensive institutional care. They have responded by investing in the potential of the interdisciplinary team to integrate medical, psychological, social, nutritional, and rehabilitative care. So far, suspicions held by skeptics that these incentives might lead to underservice of this vulnerable population are unconfirmed: rates of disenrollment from the PACE plans (5% to 6% per year) are among the lowest in the Medicare HMO industry. PACE appears to exemplify the possibility of effectively integrating the funding and the health care for the small segment of the elderly population with disability and complex health needs (Williams, 1997). Its effects on health-related outcomes and total societal costs remain to be determined.

SHMO II: The Social Health Maintenance Organization

Another experiment, the Social Health Maintenance Organization (SHMO), began in the middle 1980s. HCFA authorized the first SHMO programs, like PACE, to stimulate the delivery of flexible, integrated acute and long-term care for Medicare beneficiaries. Unlike PACE, however, the SHMO demonstrations are intended to serve not only low-income disabled seniors but the full range of older Medicare beneficiaries. They receive capitation payments equal to 100% of Medicare's AAPCC in return for covering limited long-term care services (short-term nursing home care and $7,500 to 12,000 per year for community-based care) plus the usual Medicare benefits. As with PACE, developers hoped that the resulting comprehensive coverage would lead organizations to develop integrated systems that would better promote health and functional independence and minimize undesirable and expensive events such as hospitalization and institutionalization (Kane et al., 1997). Table 16.2 shows the fundamental features of PACE and SHMO.

The four SHMO sites (in California, Minnesota, New York, and Oregon) developed systems of care that

- annually screened all enrollees to identify those at high risk
- comprehensively assessed high-risk enrollees who were living in the community and were certified as eligible for nursing home care (i.e. were nursing home certifiable, NHC)
- provided case management
- offered home- and community-based services, such as home health care, transportation, adult day care, and home keeping and personal care services

The seniors who enrolled in SHMO plans (4,000 to 7,000 per plan) received medical care that was similar to that provided in typical Medicare HMOs (Harrington, Lynch, & Newcomer, 1993). The 5% to 10% of enrollees who were NHC also received well-coordinated home- and community-based services through their case manager. Thus, SHMOs achieved the goals of integrating the funding and the social services of long-term care. They did not, however, achieve the integration of medical and social services, nor did they utilize much geriatric expertise, even for NHC enrollees (Harrington et al., 1993).

The enrollees in this first round of SHMOs experienced outcomes similar to those of the control populations; these SHMOs achieved no clear cost savings over the fee-for-service system (Harrington & Newcomer, 1991; Manton, Newcomer, Lowrimore, Vertrees, & Harrington, 1993). Based on the lessons learned, however, a new round of updated SHMOs (SHMO II) has now begun. In order to attain a greater degree of effectiveness and integration of services in SHMO II, these organizations have pledged to develop systems of care that incorporate not only the primary features of the original SHMO programs (screening, assessment, case management, transportation, and home- and community-based services) but also

- geriatric practice guidelines
- professionals with expertise in geriatrics (e.g., geriatricians and gerontological nurse practitioners)
- coordination of social and medical services
- education and incentives to help primary care providers incorporate the principles of geriatrics into their care of SHMO II patients

As a result, SHMO II will focus not only on disabled enrollees (as the SHMO I programs did) but on all enrollees with chronic illnesses or increased risk of future hospital admission or disability. To make this economically feasible, HCFA will adjust its capitation rates according to the risk status of the enrollees, paying eight times as much for those at highest risk as for those at lowest risk.

Like PACE, SHMO II is a bold experiment. Integration will inevitably face difficult challenges—developing systems that collect, manage, and communicate information and nurturing effective working relationships among primary care providers, case managers, geriatrics experts, and all of the other providers of health-related services. An extensive quasi-experimental evaluation will compare the health status, quality of life, and costs of care of the enrollees in the SHMO II with those in other Medicare HMO plans.

Programs for Dually Eligible Seniors

A third experiment in integration originated not with HCFA, but with other organizations that purchase health care for older populations. Like

TABLE 16.2   Features of the PACE and SHMO Experiments

	PACE	SHMO
Enrollees	Age 55 years or older, nursing home certifiable	Age 65 years or older
Type of services provided	Acute and long-term care	Acute and long-term care
Limits of long-term care benefits	None	$7,500 to $12,000 per year for community-based care; several weeks of NH care
Method of integration	Interdisciplinary team	Determined by sponsoring organization
Case load per site	120 to 440	4,000 to 7,000
Payers	Medicare (2.39 x AAPCC); Medicaid or copayments	Medicare (1.00 x AAPCC); Medicaid or copayments

HCFA, these organizations recognized the potential advantages of pooling Medicare and Medicaid funds to integrate acute and long-term care. Those taking the lead so far include state governments, which administer Medicaid programs, and managed care organizations that receive capitated payments from both Medicaid and Medicare. In each case, the pooled Medicaid and Medicare dollars support flexible new systems of caring for dually eligible (Medicaid-Medicare) seniors. The oldest of these programs (operated by Medica in Minneapolis) began only in 1996, so the integration of delivery systems is still rudimentary, and no evaluative data are available yet.

CONCLUSION

Even after we know the results of these experiments in care integration, restructuring our health systems will be costly and will require strong leadership, willingness to change, firm commitment, and perseverance. At this time, we cannot compel this evolution by pointing to incontrovertible proof that client-centered, integrated systems produce superior outcomes. The relevant evidence is sparse and inconsistent; we need much more information about many questions, including

- the people who need integrated services (How complex must their needs be?)
- how to integrate services (Do caregivers need to discuss cases, or will electronic databases and e-mail suffice?)
- the limits of integration (At what point are the benefits of additional services outweighed by the burden of the increased complexity of care?)
- how to share the costs and the rewards of integration (How can funders, insurers, providers, community agencies, clients, and families participate equitably?)
- the benefits of integration (Does it lead to better health, greater functional ability, lower costs, and/or more satisfied clients and providers?)
- the quality of care in capitated, integrated systems (How can we ensure that financial pressures do not lead to underservice in the name of integration?)

Despite the intuitive appeal of integrated clinical services, the present lack of definitive answers to these questions supports the health care industry's caution in seeking clinical integration. With their eyes on market share and quarterly financial reports, most organizations have been unwilling to make the sizable investments needed to achieve integration within a few years. The consolidation of insurance companies and various providers of health care under large corporate umbrellas creates some opportunities for integrating services, but the ubiquitous residual nonintegrated accounting systems present additional serious and persistent obstacles. Meanwhile, much work remains to be done to develop and refine the tools of integration: electronic data management and transfer, transfacility clinical guidelines, collaborative professional relationships, case management, client and family participation in care, and equitable arrangements for sharing financial risks and rewards.

REFERENCES

Boult, C., Boult, L., Morishita, L., Smith, S. L., & Kane, R. L. (1998). Outpatient geriatrics evaluation and management (GEM). *Journal of the American Geriatrics Society, 46*(3), 296–302.

Eng, C., Pedulla, J., Eleazer, G. P., McCann, R., & Fox, N. (1997). Program of all-inclusive care for the elderly (PACE): An innovative model of integrated geriatric care and financing. *Journal of the American Geriatrics Society, 45,* 223–232.

Fama, T., & Fox, P. (1997). Efforts to improve primary care delivery to nursing home residents. *Journal of the American Geriatrics Society, 45,* 627–632.

Harrington, C., Lynch, M., & Newcomer, R. J. (1993). Medical services in social health maintenance organizations. *Gerontologist, 33,* 790–800.

Harrington, C., & Newcomer, R. J. (1991). Social health maintenance organizations' service use and costs, 1985–1989. *Health Care Financing Review, 12,* 37–52.

Kane, R. L., Kane, R. A., Finch, M., Harrington, C., Newcomer, R., Miller, N., & Hulbert, M. (1997). S/HMOs, the second generation: Building on the experience of the first social health maintenance organization demonstrations. *Journal of the American Geriatrics Society, 45,* 101–107.

Kassirer, J. P. (1996). Mergers and acquisitions—Who benefits? Who loses? *New England Journal of Medicine, 334,* 722–723.

Landefeld, C. S., Palmer, R. M., Kresevic, D. M., Fortinsky, R. H., & Kowal, J. (1995). A randomized trial of care in a hospital medical unit especially designed to improve the functional outcomes of acutely ill older adults. *New England Journal of Medicine, 332,* 1338–1344.

Manton, K. G., Newcomer, R., Lowrimore, G. R., Vertrees, J. C., & Harrington, C. (1993). Social/health maintenance organization and fee-for-service outcomes over time. *Health Care Financing Review, 15,* 173–202.

Melin, A., Hakansson, S., & Bygren, L. (1993). The cost and effectiveness of rehabilitation in the home: A study of Swedish elderly. *American Journal of Public Health, 83,* 356–362.

Pacala, J. T., Kane, R. L., Smith, M. A., & Atherly, A. J. (1998). Quality of care in the Program of All-inclusive Care of the Elderly. *Journal of the American Geriatrics Society.* Manuscript submitted for publication.

Reuben, D. B., Borok, G. M., Wolde-Tsadik, G., Ershoff, D. H., Fishman, L. K., Ambrosini, V. L., Liu, Y., Rubenstein, L. Z., & Beck, J. C. (1995). A randomized trial of comprehensive geriatric assessment in the care of hospitalized patients. *New England Journal of Medicine, 332,* 1345–1350.

Rich, M. W., Beckham, V., Wittenberg, C., Leven, C. V., Freedland, K. E., & Carney, R. M. (1995). A multidisciplinary intervention to prevent the readmission of elderly patients with congestive heart failure. *New England Journal of Medicine, 333,* 1190–1195.

vonSternberg, T., Hepburn, K. Cibuzar, P., Convery, L., Dokken, B., Haefemeyer, J., Rettke, S., Ripley, J., Vosenau, V., Rothe, P., Schurle, D., & Won-Savage, R. (1997). Post-hospital sub-acute care: An example of a managed care model. *Journal of the American Geriatrics Society, 45,* 87–91.

Williams, T. F. (1987). Integration of geriatric assessment into the community. *Clinics in Geriatric Medicine, 3,* 111–117.

Williams, T. F. (1997). PACE: A continuing evolving success. *Journal of the American Geriatrics Society, 45,* 244.

17

The Role of the Older Person in Managing Illness

Michael Von Korff and Edward H. Wagner

INTRODUCTION

Under the best of circumstances, managing frailty and chronic illness in older persons can be complex and difficult for patients and challenging for health care providers. Beyond carrying out prescribed medical regimens, patients must monitor and manage symptoms, engage in activities that protect and promote health, and manage the impacts of illness on their daily functioning, emotions, and interpersonal relationships. These activities constitute the core tasks of caring for chronic illness (Andersen, 1992; Clark et al., 1991; Hill, Kelleher, & Shumaker, 1992).

Self-management and medical management are sometimes viewed as competing strategies for caring for illness rather than as interdependent parts of collaboration between patients and health care providers. When "self-management," "self-care," and "self-help" imply management without access to guidance or support from health care providers, these terms carry negative connotations, both to health care providers and to patients. However, geriatric care is rarely effective in the absence of adequate self-management, and self-management in the absence of appropriate medical supervision and support often yields less than optimal outcomes. Collaborative management strengthens and supports patients' abilities and self-confidence in managing their health and illnesses within a context of appropriate and effective medical care. Recent evidence has revealed that such collaborative approaches to patient care improve physiologic, emotional, and functional outcomes. Unfortunately, modern health care systems have rarely put them into practice (Lorig, 1993; Mazze, 1994; Wagner, Austin, & Von Korff, 1996).

This chapter summarizes scientific evidence regarding interventions that support the patient's role in the provision of care. It then identifies elements essential for achieving productive interactions between patients and health care providers and concludes by identifying patient, provider, and system barriers that impede the development of such collaboration.

SELF-MANAGEMENT DEFINED

Patients and their families are the primary providers of care for chronic health problems (Clark et al., 1991; Lorig, 1993; Sobel, 1995). Accordingly, health care systems need to strengthen and support the abilities of older patients and their families to maximize independence and functioning, prevent frailty and disease, and manage chronic illnesses. As defined in chapter 3, self-management encompasses

- engaging in activities that promote health and build physiologic reserve—for example, exercising, eating nutritious food, avoiding tobacco, participating in social activities, and getting enough sleep
- interacting with health care professionals and systems and adhering to recommended prevention and treatment protocols
- monitoring one's own physical and emotional status, using the results to make appropriate management decisions
- managing the impacts of illness on one's emotions, self-esteem, relations with others, and ability to function in important roles

(Clark et al., 1991, 1992; Lorig, 1993; Wagner et al., 1996). Unfortunately, the training of health care workers, the organization of health care services, and the traditional expectations of patients often stand in the way of effective self-management.

For the most part, this chapter focuses on individual patients. Increasingly, however, health systems are looking to patient groups for guidance in program development and operations, using focus groups, surveys, and forums among patients and families with particular care needs. This trend in population-level self-management could be a valuable development if structurally incorporated into an organizational decision-making process.

EVIDENCE ABOUT INTERVENTIONS THAT STRENGTHEN THE PATIENT'S ROLE

Care of the older person that minimizes frailty and the complications of chronic disease requires an organized and planned approach to management. It requires active involvement of and communication among patient, caregiver, and professionals, which explains our preference for the term *collaborative management.* Patients with chronic problems benefit when they are engaged in care that helps them identify problems, plan for problems that are likely to be most significant, and carry out plans to manage targeted problems (Andersen, 1992; Clark et al., 1992; Lorig, Laurin, & Holman, 1984).

Enhancing Patients' Involvement in Their Care

Across a variety of chronic conditions, interventions that enhance the involvement and skills of patients have led to improvements in disease severity, daily functioning, emotional well-being, adherence to medical treatments, control of pain and other symptoms, confidence in one's ability to manage illness, and health care utilization and costs. Most self-management interventions focus on the knowledge and skills required for the patient and family to monitor and manage the condition. Although traditional patient education programs also emphasize knowledge acquisition, they tend to reinforce the primacy of professional decision-making by accentuating patient compliance with prescribed regimens. These programs generally are ineffective. More successful interventions attempt to enhance "patient empowerment" (Anderson et al., 1995), "patient activation," or "patient participation." These concepts posit that care and health outcomes will improve when patients make informed choices about their health, life-style, and health care and share decision-making about illness and illness care with health professionals. Self-efficacy, the confidence that one can perform important behaviors, is a critical intermediate outcome for these programs. Several specific interventions have been shown to increase self-efficacy and participation in care and improve health and utilization outcomes (Anderson et al., 1995; Giloth, 1990; Greenfield, Kaplan, Ware, Yano, & Frank, 1988).

A growing body of evidence suggests that self-management is most effective when patients ask questions, express preferences, and solicit information (Delbanco & Daley, 1996). Health care providers often need to promote these behaviors, especially in older persons accustomed to more authoritarian physicians. In a now classic randomized trial, Greenfield and colleagues (1988) found that diabetic patients who were prepared for their clinic visits in advance were more able to elicit important information from their doctors. In preparing, patients interacted in the waiting room for 15 minutes with a nonphysician research assistant, who gave specific advice about asking questions about the physician's approach to diabetes. In follow-up, the prepared patients showed more favorable glycosated hemoglobin levels than the control patients (who had received traditional patient education). Although intervention patients asked more questions than did control patients, physicians could not discern which patients received the intervention.

Anderson and colleagues (1995) have developed a set of counseling techniques intended to "empower" patients, making them more confident and competent managers of their illness. The techniques, usually applied by nurse educators, emphasize listening, referring problems back to the patient for solutions, and constantly reinforcing the patient's role and successes in self-management. A wait-list randomized trial with diabetic patients compared the empowerment approach with conventional patient education. Patients receiving the empowerment intervention had higher levels of self-efficacy and better glucose control.

Assessment

Clinical assessment can facilitate self-management if it includes, in addition to the patient's medical condition and functional status, information about the patient's preferences for treatment and the psychological and physical resources that the patient and his or her family can dedicate to chronic illness management. Assessment can help care providers (1) understand the patient's life situation and preferences, (2) match treatment recommendations to the individual patient's needs and preferences, and (3) shift the emphasis from responding to the patient's complaints and crises to collaborative monitoring and preventing adverse sequelae. Planning an effective care strategy can then take these factors into account. Too often, however, geriatric assessment is viewed more narrowly as a method of finding high-cost, high-risk subjects and referring them for special interventions.

Although questionnaires can be efficient in obtaining information, integrating questionnaire-based assessment into routine health care delivery has been difficult. One group has attempted to integrate office-based assessment into the routine primary care of older adults by using a bar-coded questionnaire and an electronic information system. At each visit, the patient completes a brief questionnaire about his or her health, functional status, and satisfaction with care. Bar-coded questionnaires are scanned into a computer that processes the patient's responses and generates a flow sheet with reminders for the physician and a letter with suggestions for the patient. A randomized trial found that patients who participated in this program received better care and were more satisfied with their care (Wasson, Jette, Johnson, Mohr, & Nelson, 1997).

COLLABORATIVE TREATMENT PLANNING

Across a wide range of effective chronic disease and geriatric interventions, the crucial step following assessment is for the provider team and the patient (and family) to define the problems to be managed (Clark, Janz, Dodge, & Sharpe, 1992; Giloth, 1990; Inui & Carter, 1985). Providers tend to define problems in terms of abnormal laboratory tests or specific diagnoses. Patients and families often emphasize inability to perform valued activities, discontent, incontinence, falling, loneliness, or treatment side effects. Patients are likely to benefit when these two perspectives are harmonized.

Several techniques have been applied to the process of collaborative problem definition. Collaborative treatment planning requires a provider who is willing and able to listen to patient concerns, provide useful information, and share decision-making responsibilities. The evidence suggests that older patients are more satisfied and adherent to recommended therapy when their providers are less authoritarian and more participatory. Some evidence also suggests that providers can change their approach to communicating with patients through training (Miller & Rollnick, 1991). One study found that, among physicians involved in the Medical Outcomes Study (MOS), those who had received training in interviewing were more likely to involve patients in decision-making (Kaplan, Greenfield, Gandek, Rogers, & Ware, 1996). Further, the patients of those MOS physicians rated as most participatory were half as likely to change physicians in the next year and significantly more satisfied with their care than patients who rated their physicians as least participatory. Other simple techniques for increasing patient input have proven to be effective. Teaching doctors to ask simple questions like "What is the most difficult part of managing your illness?" can help in identifying patient problems missed in a traditional clinical interview (Glasgow, 1995; Inui & Carter, 1985). Brief questionnaires can also help assess and prioritize problems and assess readiness for self-management tasks; they can form a basis for giving patients personalized feedback on self-management (Montgomery, Lieberman, Singh, & Fries, 1994).

After years of receiving paternalistic health care, many older patients are not prepared to be active participants in their care; they too may need training. One particularly cost-effective approach uses groups to help patients target problems, set goals, and plan care (Andersen, 1992; Lorig & Holman, 1993). Traditionally, groups have been organized for patients with a single condition (e.g., arthritis or breast cancer), limiting their feasibility in primary-care settings, because few problems affect a sufficient number of patients to constitute a group. Recently, a self-management training group that combined patients with different chronic conditions produced positive results (Leveille et al., submitted; Lorig et al., 1994). This approach to managing generic chronic illness could boost the feasibility of using group interventions in primary-care settings.

Once patient and provider have agreed about which problems are significant, they must target the most important problem, set goals for addressing that problem, and develop an action plan (Clark et al., 1992; Glasgow, 1995). There is growing consensus that targeting should be based both on the significance of the problem and on the patient's motivation and readiness to address the problem (Ruggiero & Prochaska, 1993). In many successful interventions, nurse educators have facilitated the processes of targeting, goal setting, planning, and implementing (DeBusk et al., 1994; Rich et al., 1995; Stuck et al., 1995).

Self-Management Training and Support

Self-management training refers to educational and behavior-change interventions that enhance the knowledge, skills, confidence, and problem-solving abilities of patients who are managing their health problems. Self-management training may be broad in scope, covering the full range of self-management tasks, or focused, such as an exercise program. Individual and group instruction are effective for self-management training and support (Arseneau, Mason, Wood, Schwab, & Green, 1994; Fawzy et al., 1990; Gilden, Hendryx, Clar, Casia, & Singh, 1992). Home-based instruction, in which patients receive high-quality instructional materials along with personalized feedback (delivered by telephone or through the mail), is a promising, low-cost strategy for supporting self-management. Such an approach has resulted in improved function for patients with Parkinson's disease, as described in chapter 3 (Montgomery et al., 1994), and reduced risk factors for coronary heart disease in patients with myocardial infarctions (DeBusk et al., 1994). Computer-based instruction in self-management is another emerging possibility (Glasgow, Toobert, & Hampson, 1996). In this case, the medium may be less important than the message.

As mentioned earlier, it is important that self-management training experiences be individualized, based on each patient's motivation and readiness, and aligned with priorities agreed upon by patient and provider. Thus, self-management training may be most effective if organized as a continuing set of experiences in which the sequence and pace of learning match the individuals' needs, abilities, motivation level, and preferences. For example, Glasgow (1995) has advocated low-intensity self-management interventions for all diabetics in a population, reserving more expensive and intensive interventions for appropriately targeted, higher-risk patients. This approach seems preferable to time-limited patient education programs offered only at the time of diagnosis.

Sustained Follow-up

Follow-up should occur at consistent and clearly defined intervals. At these "checkpoints," providers can obtain key information on medical and functional status, identify potential complications at an early stage, check progress toward implementation of the management plan, make necessary modifications to the management plan, and reinforce patients' efforts. Such follow-up can be accomplished by scheduled visits, telephone calls, electronic mail, or mailed reminders or questionnaires (DeBusk et al., 1994; Glasgow, 1995; Gruesser, Bott, Ellermann, Kronsbein, & Joergens, 1993; Holman, Lubeck, Dutton, & Brown, 1988; Katon et al., 1995; Stuck et al., 1995). In several randomized trials, ongoing telephone contact proved to be a highly effective method of follow-up (Wasson et al., 1992; Weinberger et al., 1995). For example, DeBusk and colleagues (1994) randomly assigned coronary artery disease patients to usual care or to physician-directed, nurse-provided case management for modification of risk factors. The intervention patients received follow-up after hospital discharge primarily by telephone. Relative to usual care, the intervention favorably affected smoking cessation, cholesterol levels, and functional status.

Collaborative Problem-Solving

Interventions that strengthen and support self-management follow theories of social learning and self-regulation (Clark et al., 1992; Glasgow & Osteen, 1992; Lorig & Holman, 1993; Schulz & Williamson, 1993). A key principle is that patients must become informed and active problem-solvers with respect to their health and must respond to the changes in their diseases, symptoms, emotions, and life circumstances that influence functioning. The interventions tested in randomized controlled trials typically provided a well-defined structure within which patients learned to manage and adapt to chronic illness. Specific problem-solving interventions usually include identifying an illness-related problem that the patient is motivated to resolve, setting specific goals related to solving the problem, identifying various ways to reach the goal and the barriers to reaching it, assessing the pros and cons of various solutions and choosing one that is promising, making a commitment and putting the plan into action, checking on progress and making midcourse corrections as needed, and rewarding effort and progress toward achieving goals (Clark et al., 1992). This problem-solving approach provides patients with a framework for applying their life experiences and skills to the challenges they face in managing chronic illness.

For example, Clark and colleagues (1992) evaluated an 8-hour group intervention for patients 60 years and older with heart disease. The program focused on "self-regulation," the patient's ability to identify, research, and resolve problems confronted in the self- or medical management of heart disease. Among the problems considered by the group were those related to communicating with health professionals. One year later, patients randomized to receive the intervention who attended one or more group sessions reported higher self-efficacy and better health status, particularly in psychosocial dimensions.

Individualizing Treatment Approaches

Treatment plans should align with the clinical, behavioral, and cultural characteristics of individual patients. In a recent literature review, Delbanco and Daley (1996) found that providers' efforts to elicit patients' preferences and involve them in treatment planning and decision-making consistently increased patient satisfaction, adherence, and outcomes. Interventions are more likely to be effective when matched to what a patient feels ready to handle. One study tested a computer-based approach to dietary counseling that tailored the messages to diabetic patients' readiness to change (Prochaska & DiClemente, 1983), self-efficacy, and perceived barriers to change. Patients randomized to the intervention group reduced their total serum cholesterol levels by an average of 9 mg/dl, while control subjects, who received usual care, experienced a small increase in total cholesterol (Glasgow et al., 1996).

Recent work has also demonstrated that individuals vary widely in their preferences for treatment and, perhaps more importantly, for different outcomes. Benign prostatic hyperplasia (BPH) is a nearly inevitable accompaniment of aging, and a host of surgical and nonsurgical treatments now exist. There is considerable variation in how older men rate the importance of BPH symptoms (e.g., nocturia) and treatment side effects (e.g., postsurgical impotence) (Fowler et al., 1988), and these ratings affect their decision-making about therapy (Barry, Fowler, Mulley, Henderson, & Wennberg, 1995). For example, older men for whom sexual activity is still very important were less likely to choose surgery, while men who viewed their urinary symptoms as particularly troublesome were more likely to choose surgery. Barry and colleagues used interactive computer-videodisc technology to elicit patients' clinical characteristics and preferences and to provide tailored information about the benefits and risks of various treatment options using patient testimonials. Patients assigned to the interactive video were significantly more satisfied with their decision.

BARRIERS TO ENHANCED COLLABORATION BETWEEN PATIENTS AND PROVIDERS

Despite mounting evidence of their effectiveness, self-management and patient activation interventions have not been widely integrated into routine health care for older patients. Patient, provider, and system barriers impede their integration into routine health care.

Patient Barriers

The cumulative burdens of chronic illness and loss of function may impair a patient's ability and readiness to engage in self-management. Some chronic illnesses are accompanied by pain and fatigue that can undermine motivation and self-confidence (Andersen, 1992). Emotional reactions may include anger, worry, a sense of loss, feelings that one's body or basic health is failing, or denial that anything is wrong or has changed. Among older adults, repeated losses and accompanying depressive symptoms, which are common, may diminish the self-efficacy required for effective self-management.

The skills required to take care of a chronic illness require time to develop and effort to sustain. Patients often prematurely terminate long-term medical treatments, such as taking medicines, because they perceive that the potential benefits are not worth the side effects and hassles (Haynes, Taylor, & Sackett, 1979). A frequent response to illness is to take it easy and rest.

Social support is also important for people who are managing chronic illness. Support from family and friends generally has positive effects, but not always. Family members may inadvertently undermine a patient's efforts to adhere to dietary changes, exercise regimens, or medication regimens (Burg & Seeman, 1994; Schafer, McCaul, & Glasgow, 1986). They may also relieve the patient of too many responsibilities, contributing to deactivation (Clark, Janz, Dodge, & Garrity, 1994).

Patients are often poorly prepared for getting what they need from health care providers. They may be reluctant to ask even basic questions about how to manage illness, or to ask for clarification when they do not understand the information provided (Anderson et al., 1995; Giloth, 1990; Greenfield et al., 1988). This reflects a broader problem of providers expecting and patients assuming a passive stance (Wallerstein, 1992). This phenomenon may be especially prevalent among older persons. The patient-activating interventions described above may help to overcome such reticence.

Provider Barriers

The traditions of medicine have emphasized diagnosis and curative treatment of acute conditions (McCormick & Inui, 1992; Wagner et al., 1996). These traditions have fostered the management of the symptoms, activity limitations, and health crises of old patients as if they were a series of acute events. As a result, care of frailty and chronic illness is often reactive, unplanned, and unscheduled; patients and their families do not receive essential services that educate, train, and support them (Sobel, 1995).

During health care encounters, providers rarely ask older patients to share their understanding of their illness or to identify their goals for managing the illness (Connelly, 1987; Smith & Hoppe, 1991). Moreover, while maintaining adequate performance of important roles (e.g., parent, grandparent, spouse, breadwinner, and athlete) is a high priority for most older persons, providers, trained and accustomed to responding to signs and symptoms, do not consistently ask patients about the effects of health-related problems on their ability to function in these roles. When providers do discuss functional problems, they are often poorly prepared to help patients find solutions (Sobel, 1995). Randomized trials have tested the value of collecting functional status information from patients and reporting it to their physicians. This intervention had but a minimal impact on treatment choices or other elements of care (Calkins et al., 1994; Rubenstein et al., 1989). The most likely explanation is that many physicians simply do not know how to respond to functional deficits. The focus of the medical encounter remains on evaluating and treating medical problems, even when functional problems may be more important to the patient and to the ultimate outcome of the illness.

Perhaps because physicians view themselves as the primary influence on the outcomes of their patients' illnesses (albeit in collaboration with the patient), they rarely offer their patients opportunities to share experiences with and learn from other patients (Ruberman, 1992). Patients have few chances to talk about the fears and frustrations, the pain and fatigue, the anger and loss of control that can accompany aging. As a result, many practical, effective ways of coping with the effects of illness are not communicated to patients. Although patients benefit from support groups in which they have structured opportunities to discuss emotional reactions to illness and to develop skills for coping with illness (Fawzy et al., 1990; Spiegel, Bloom, Kraemer, & Gottheil, 1989), routine health care rarely incorporates such services. The Cooperative Health Care Clinic, described in chapter 3, illustrates the salutary impact of combining clinical care and a support group experience in the same clinic visit (Beck et al., 1997).

Deficiencies in follow-up stand out as another significant barrier to self-management (Wagner et al., 1996). Follow-up that is triggered only by acute illness, bothersome symptoms, treatment side effects, and patients' worries contains little time for reinventing self-management.

System Barriers

Providers Rarely Integrate Patient Self-Management or Activation Interventions Into Everyday Practice. The prescription of self-management interventions such as disease-management training programs, support groups, or supervised exercise is unusual. Most practices do not have a reliable referral path to self-management training and support. In contrast, current health care systems have incorporated links to support services for the delivery of medical interventions (e.g., drugs, testing services, medical procedures, and physical therapy) so that these interventions can be readily prescribed by physicians and reliably delivered to patients.

Office Visits Are the Focus of Care.   The organization of primary medical care around the brief office visit is a critical impediment to enhancing the patient's role in care. Abandoning the 10 to 20-minute office visit as the basic unit of health care could lead to improved and more collaborative geriatric care. Alternative "cooperative health care clinics" (Beck et al., 1997) or "mini-clinics" (Thorn & Russell, 1973), in which provider teams see groups of senior patients with similar conditions, increase the time and opportunities for patient participation and self-management support.

Scheduled telephone contact is more effective and less costly for routine follow-up of chronic illness than unscheduled and unplanned office visits (Holman et al., 1998; Renee, Weinberger, Mazzuca, Brandt, & Katz, 1992; van Elderen-van Kemendade et al., 1994; Wasson et al., 1992). For example, in a sample of elderly male patients with chronic disease, Wasson and colleagues (1992) evaluated the effects of making regular telephone contact while doubling the recommended interval between visits. Relative to controls, patients with telephone care had fewer clinic visits, both scheduled and unscheduled; they also used less medication and less inpatient care than controls. Among patients with fair to poor health at baseline, telephone care was also associated with significantly favorable effects on physical functioning. As documented in this chapter and throughout this book, practice-initiated telephone follow-up is a hallmark of many successful interventions and is becoming an integral component of modern evidence-based geriatric care.

Health Care Systems Fail to Realize the Full Potential of Allied Health Professionals.   While many believe that allied health professionals (e.g., nurses, physician assistants, and social workers) should play a central role in geriatric care, health care systems often engage them in managing acute primary care or serving as peripheral consultants. As part of national health care in Germany, office nurses have been trained and funded to provide self-management support to patients with diabetes and hypertension. Randomized trials examining this approach have demonstrated improved glucose and blood pressure control (Gruesser et al., 1993). It is often difficult to integrate allied health professionals into service delivery arrangements, however, when reimbursement or "productivity" assessment is tied to the number of patients seen and/or the number of procedures performed by physicians.

Primary and Specialty Care Lack Cooperative Coordination. The positive results associated with successful geriatric evaluation and management programs point to the importance of geriatric expertise and experience in maximizing outcomes for older patients. While close collaboration between primary care, specialty care, and patients would appear to be beneficial, primary care and specialty care generally tend to be poorly integrated, confusing patients and undermining their role in managing their health. Various attempts to contribute geriatric advice and consultation to providers of primary care to ambulatory older patients (outpatient geriatric assessment and consultation clinics) have produced mixed results, as others have discussed elsewhere in this book. Reuben and colleagues (1996) posited that the success of outpatient geriatric consultation might well depend on the nature of the communication between consultation team, primary care provider, and patient. Based on focus groups of primary care physicians and the literature on physician behavior change, they augmented the usual consultation note with a telephone call and copies of the recommendations and relevant published articles from the geriatrician to the patient's primary physician. In addition, they shared the results of the consultation with the patient through telephone calls and written materials. This two-pronged approach produced rates of implementation of recommendations by both physicians and patients that were as high as or higher than those previously reported from consultation units. Experiences like this suggest four important elements for improving coordination of care between specialty and primary care:

1. The roles of all parties, including the patient, should be clearly understood.
2. Communication between specialist and generalist should be interactive.
3. Evidence of effectiveness should accompany specialists' recommendations to generalists.
4. Specialists' recommendations should be shared with patients.

Support From Information Systems Is Inadequate. Information systems can play a critical role in improving the management of chronic illness and in increasing patients' involvement in their care (Wagner et al., 1996). In the absence of adequate information system support, health care providers have difficulty ensuring that patients receive preventive and health-maintaining services on a timely basis or providing sustained support for patients who are carrying out long-term management plans. At present, ambulatory-care information systems are not widely used to support collaborative management functions, such as identifying patients with specific chronic conditions; developing and recording management plans; monitoring implementation of management plans; monitoring physiologic, symptomatic, and functional outcomes; or reminding providers or patients when lapses in performance occur. The use of new computer systems that engage directly with patients has drawn intense interest (Barry et al., 1995; Glasgow et al., 1996). These systems can potentially collect and share patient data with all members of the practice team in real time.

Significant Financial Barriers Also Impede the Implementation of Self-Management Interventions.   Although self-management interventions are often inexpensive, they sometimes require the participation of providers who are not reimbursed, or they call for behavior-change services not presently covered by insurance.

Health Care Systems Have Poorly Developed Links With Community Resources.   Although many communities have resources that could enhance self-management, few health care systems have developed relationships for tapping into and helping shape those resources (see chapter 16). Linkages between health care settings and community resources are the exception rather than the rule. Senior centers, for example, could play a role in providing self-management training and support services for elderly people with chronic illness, but working ties with primary care providers would need to develop. Voluntary organizations (e.g., the American Diabetes Association, the American Heart Association, the Alzheimer's Association, and the Arthritis Foundation) could also help provide self-management training and support services in conjunction with primary health care clinics, but they rarely do so. Even in health care systems with established health education departments, the links between community self-management training services and primary health care are often tenuous.

SUMMARY

Excellent geriatric care recognizes the crucial role of patient and family in determining outcomes. It ensures that patient needs and concerns are routinely elicited, that patients and providers collaborate in clinical and self-management, and that interventions are tailored to the preferences of patients and caregivers. Until recently, most health systems and provider groups have paid scant attention to patients' self-management potential and their role in making decisions about their care. Ignoring advanced directives at the end of life is but one manifestation. The evidence suggests that optimizing health outcomes will depend on the implementation of effective interventions that enhance patient participation in the collaborative management of frailty and chronic illnesses. Developing these new collaborative relationships between older persons and health care providers and health systems is a major challenge facing organized health care systems.

REFERENCES

Andersen, B. L. (1992). Psychological interventions for cancer patients to enhance the quality of life. *Journal of Consulting & Clinical Psychology, 60,* 552–568.

Anderson, R. M., Funnell, M. M., Butler, P. M., Arnold, M. S., Fitzgerald, J. T., & Feste, C. C. (1995). Patient empowerment: Results of a randomized controlled trial. *Diabetes Care, 18,* 943–949.

Arseneau, D. L., Mason, A. C., Wood, O. B., Schwab, E., & Green, D. (1994). A comparison of learning activity packages and classroom instruction for diet management of patients with non-insulin-dependent diabetes mellitus. *Diabetes Education, 20,* 509–514.

Barry, M. J., Fowler, F. J., Mulley, A. G., Henderson, J. V. Jr., & Wennberg, J. E. (1995). Patient reactions to a program designed to facilitate patient participation in treatment decisions for benign prostatic hyperplasia. *Medical Care, 33,* 771–782.

Beck, A., Scott, J., Williams, P., Robertson, B., Jackson, D., Gade, G., & Cowan, P. (1997). A randomized trail of group outpatient visits for chronically ill older HMO members: The cooperative health care clinic. *Journal of the American Geriatrics Society, 45,* 543–549.

Burg, M. M., Seeman, T. E. (1994). Families and health: The negative side of social ties. *Annals of Behavioral Medicine, 16,* 109–115.

Calkins, D. R., Rubenstein, L. V., Cleary, P. D., Davies, A. R., Jette, A. M., Fink, A., Kosecoff, J., Young, R. T., Brook, R. H., & Delbanco, T. L. (1994). Functional disability screening of ambulatory patients: A randomized controlled trial in a hospital-based group practice. *Journal of General Internal Medicine, 9,* 590–592.

Clark, N. M., Becker, M. H., Janz, N. K., Lorig, K., Rakowski, W., & Anderson, L. (1991). Self-management of chronic disease by older adults: A review and questions for research. *Journal of Aging and Health, 3,* 3–27.

Clark, N. M., Janz, N. K., Becker, M. H., Schork, M. A., Wheeler, J., Liang, J., Dodge, J. A., Keteyian, S., Rhoads, K. L., & Santinga, J. T. (1992). Impact of self-management education on the functional health status of older adults with heart disease. *Gerontologist, 32,* 438–443.

Clark, N. M., Janz, N. K., Dodge, J. A., & Garrity, C. R. (1994). Managing heart disease: A study of the experiences of older women. *Journal of the American Medical Women's Association, 49,* 202–206.

Clark, N. M., Janz, N. K., Dodge, J. A., & Sharpe, P. A. (1992). Self-regulation of health behavior: The "take PRIDE" program. *Health-Education Quarterly, 19,* 341–354.

Connelly. C. E. (1987). Self-care and the chronically ill patient. *Nursing Clinics of North America, 22,* 621–629.

DeBusk, R. F., Miller, N. H., Superko, H. R., Dennis, C. A., Thomas, R. J., Lew, H. T., Berger, W. E., Heller, R. S., Rompf, J., Gee, D., Kraemer, H. C., Bandura, A., Ghandour, G., Clark, M., Shah, R. V., Fisher, L., & Taylor, C. B. (1994). A case-management system for coronary risk factor modification after acute myocardial infarction [comments]. *Annals of Internal Medicine, 120,* 721–729.

Delbanco, T. L., & Daley, J. (1996). Through the patient's eyes: strategies toward more successful contraception. *Obstetrics and Gynecology, 88* (supp. 3), 415–475.

Fawzy, F. I., Cousins, N., Fawzy, N. W., Kemeny, M. E., Elashoff, R., & Morton, D. (1990). A structured psychiatric intervention for cancer patients: Part 1 Changes over time in methods of coping and affective disturbance. *Archives of General Psychiatry, 47,* 720–725.

Fowler, F. J., Wennberg, J. E., Timothy, R. P., Barry, M. J., Mulley, A. G., & Hanley, D. (1988). Symptom status and quality of life following prostatectomy. *Journal of the American Medical Association, 259,* 3018–3022.

Gilden, J. L., Hendryx, M. S., Clar, S., Casia, C., & Singh, S. P. (1992). Diabetes support groups improve health care of older diabetic patients. *Journal of the American Geriatrics Society, 40,* 147–150.

Giloth, B. E. (1990). Promoting patient involvement: Educational, organizational, and environmental strategies. *Patient Education Counseling, 15,* 29–38.

Glasgow, R. E. (1995). A practical model of diabetes management and education. *Diabetes Care, 18,* 117–126.

Glasgow, R. E., & Osteen, V. L. (1992). Evaluating diabetes education: Are we measuring the most important outcomes? *Diabetes Care, 15,* 1423–1432.

Glasgow, R. E., Toobert, D. J., & Hampson, S. E. (1996). Effects of a brief, office-based intervention to facilitate diabetes dietary self-management. *Diabetes Care, 19,* 835–842.

Greenfield, S., Kaplan, S. H., Ware, J. E., Yano, E. M., & Frank, H. J. (1988). Patients' participation in medical care: Effects on blood sugar control and quality of life in diabetes. *Journal of General Internal Medicine, 3,* 448–457.

Gruesser, M., Bott, U., Ellermann, P., Kronsbein, P., & Joergens, V. (1993). Evaluation of a structured treatment and teaching program for non-insulin treated type II diabetic outpatients in Germany after the nationwide introduction of reimbursement policy for physicians. *Diabetes Care, 16,* 1268–1275.

Haynes, R. B, Taylor, D. W., & Sackett, D. L. (1979). *Compliance in health care.* Baltimore: Johns Hopkins University Press.

Hill, D. R., Kelleher, K., & Shumaker, S. A. (1992). Psychosocial interventions in adult patients with coronary heart disease and cancer: A literature review. *General Hospital Psychiatry, 14,* 28S–42S.

Holman, H., Lubeck, D., Dutton, D., & Brown, B. W. (1988). Improving health service performance by modifying medical practices. *Transactions of the Association of American Physicians, 101,* 173–179.

Inui, T. S., & Carter, W. B. (1985). Problems and prospects for health services research on provider-patient communication. *Medical Care, 23,* 521–538.

Kaplan, S., Greenfield, S., Gandek, B., Rogers, W. H., & Ware, J. E., Jr. (1996). Characteristics of physicians with participatory decision-making styles. *Annals of Internal Medicine, 124,* 497–504.

Katon, W., VonKorff, M., Lin, E., Walker, E., Simon, G. E., Bush, T., Robinson, P., & Russo, J. (1995). Collaborative management to achieve treatment guidelines. Impact on depression in primary care. *Journal of the American Medical Association, 273,* 1026–1031.

Leveille, S. G., Wagner, E. H., Davis, C., Grothaus, L., Wallace, J., LoGerfo, M., & Kent, D. Preventing disability and managing chronic illness in frail older adults: A randomized trial of a community-based partnership with primary care. Manuscript under review.

Lorig, K., Holman, H., Sobel, D., Laurenti D., Gonzalez, V., & Minor, M. (1994). Living a healthy life with chronic conditions. Palo Alto: Bull Publishing.

Lorig, K., & Holman, H. (1993). Arthritis self-management studies: A twelve-year review. *Health-Education Quarterly, 20,* 17–28.

Lorig, K., Laurin, J., & Holman, H. R. (1984). Arthritis self-management: A study of the effectiveness of patient education for the elderly. *Gerontologist, 24,* 455–457.

Lorig, K. (1993). Self-management of chronic illness: A model for the future. *Generations, 17,* 11–14.

Mazze, R. S. (1994). A systems approach to diabetes care. *Diabetes Care, 17* (Supp. 1), 5–11.

McCormick, W. C., & Inui, T. S. (1992). Geriatric preventive care: Counseling techniques in practice settings. *Clinics in Geriatric Medicine, 8,* 215–228.

Miller, W. R., & Rollnick, S. (1991). *Motivational interviewing: Preparing people to change addictive behavior.* New York: Guilford Press.

Montgomery, E. B. J., Lieberman, A., Singh, G., & Fries, J. F. (1994). Patient education and health promotion can be effective in Parkinson's disease: A randomized controlled trial [see comments]. *American Journal of Medicine, 97,* 429–435.

Prochaska, J. O., & DiClemente, C. C. (1983). Stages and processes of self-change of smoking: Toward an integrative model of change. *Journal of Consulting and Clinical Psychology, 51,* 390–395.

Renee, J., Weinberger, M., Mazzuca, S. A., Brandt, K. D., & Katz, B. P. (1992). Reduction of joint pain in patients with knee osteoarthritis who have received monthly telephone calls from lay personnel and whose medical treatment regimens have remained stable. *Arthritis and Rheumatism, 35,* 511–515.

Reuben, D. B., Maly, R. C., Hirsch, S. H., Frank, J. C., Oakes, A. M., Siu, A. L., & Hays, R. D. (1996). Physician implementation of and patient adherence to recommendations from comprehensive geriatric assessment. *American Journal of Medicine, 100,* 444–451.

Rich, M. W., Beckham, V., Wittenberg, C., Leven, C. L., Freedland, K. E., & Carney, R. M. (1995). A multidisciplinary intervention to prevent the readmission of elderly patients with congestive heart failure. *New England Journal of Medicine, 333,* 1190–1195.

Rubenstein L. V., Calkins, D. R., Young, R. T., Cleary, P. D., Fink, A., Rosecoff, J., Jette, A. M., Davies, A. R., Delbanco, T. L., & Brook, R. H. (1989). Improving patient function: A randomized trial of functional disability screening. *Annals of Internal Medicine, 111,* 836–842.

Ruberman, W. (1992). Psychosocial influences on mortality of patients with coronary heart disease [editorial; comment]. _Journal of the American Medical Association, 267_, 559–560.

Ruggiero, L., & Prochaska, J. O. (1993). Readiness for change: Application of the transtheoretical model to diabetes. _Diabetes Spectrum, 6_, 22–24.

Schafer, L. C., McCaul, K. D., & Glasgow, R. E. (1986). Supportive and nonsupportive family behaviors: Relationships to adherence and metabolic control in persons with type I diabetes. _Diabetes Care, 9_, 179–185.

Schulz, R., & Williamson, G. M. (1993). Psychosocial and behavioral dimensions of physical frailty. _Journal of Gerontology, 48_ 39–43.

Smith, R. C., & Hoppe, R. B. (1991). The patient's story: Integrating the patient- and physician-centered approaches to interviewing [comments]. _Annals of Internal Medicine, 115_, 470–477.

Sobel, D. S. (1995). Rethinking medicine: Improving health outcomes with cost-effective psychosocial interventions. _Psychosomatic Medicine, 57_, 234–244.

Spiegel, D., Bloom, J. R., Kraemer, H. C., & Gottheil, E. (1989). Effect of psychosocial treatment on survival of patients with metastatic breast cancer [comments]. _Lancet, 2_, 888–891.

Stuck, A. E., Aronow, H. U., Steiner, A., Alessi, C. A., Bula, C. J., Gold, M. N., Yuhas, K. E., Nisenbaum, R., Rubenstein, L. Z., & Beck, J. C. (1995). A trial of annual in-home comprehensive geriatric assessments for elderly people living in the community. _New England Journal of Medicine, 333_, 1184–1189.

Thorn, P. A., & Russell, R. G. (1973). Diabetic clinics today and tomorrow: Mini-clinics in general practice. _British Medical Journal, 2_, 534–536.

van Elderen-van Kemenade, T., Maes, S., & van den Broek, Y. (1994). Effects of a health education programme with telephone follow-up during cardiac rehabilitation. _British Journal of Clinical Psychology, 33_, 367–378.

Wagner, E. H., Austin, B. T., & Von Korff, M. (1996). Organizing care for patients with chronic illness. _Milbank Quarterly, 74_, 511–544.

Wallerstein N. (1992). Powerlessness, empowerment, and health: Implications for health promotion programs. _American Journal of Health Promotion, 6_, 197–205.

Wasson, J., Gaudette, C., Whaley, F., Sauvigne, A., Baribeau, P., & Welch, H. G. (1992). Telephone care as a substitute for routine clinic follow-up [comments]. _Journal of the American Medical Association, 267_, 1788–1793.

Wasson, J. H., Jette, A. M., Johnson, D. J., Mohr, J. J., & Nelson, E. C. (1997). A replicable and customizable approach to improve ambulatory care and research. _Journal of Ambulatory Care Management, 20_, 17–27.

Weinberger, M., Kirkman, M. S., Samsa, G. P., Shortliffe, E. A., Landsman, P. B., Cowper, P. A., Simel, D. L., & Feussner, J. R. (1995). A nurse-coordinated intervention for primary care patients with non-insulin-dependent diabetes mellitus: Impact on glycemic control and health-related quality of life. _Journal of General Internal Medicine 10_, 59–66.

18

Medicare and Managed Care

Harold S. Luft

INTRODUCTION

As the Medicare program enters its fourth decade, it is increasingly likely that major changes will be made in how it functions. Debates have begun to address its long-term restructuring to deal with the impending pressures of baby boomers in the second and third decades of the 21st century. The budget decisions of 1997 have incorporated short-term changes. Regardless of the details, Medicare clearly has moved a long way from the initial legislation that prohibited government interference with the practice of medicine (Social Security Act of 1965, Title XVIII, Section 1801).

In some ways, Medicare has been a leader in the managed care revolution in the United States; in other ways, it has lagged. However, because Medicare accounts for roughly 30% of all expenditures for hospital care and 20% for physician services, any changes in the Medicare program will have an enormous impact on the overall system. Moreover, as the largest single purchaser of medical care, the uniform nature of the program carries much more weight than the Medicaid programs run individually by the states, although with some federal support.

I stress in this chapter, however, that focusing just on Medicare and managed care is likely to give a distorted picture, because Medicare is rarely the only source of coverage for its beneficiaries, and its effects on the medical care system influence and are influenced by non-Medicare factors. Because the federal perspective often focuses only on the pieces of the puzzle for which it is responsible and for which it has data, the policy discussion is often incomplete. Due to the lack of data and comprehensive research, this chapter will also be incomplete, but it will hopefully lead others to pursue a more complete understanding.

This chapter first offers some brief definitions of managed care in the context of the Medicare population. It then provides an overview of enrollment trends and patterns of coverage. Risk selection is a crucial problem in the Medicare program with implications not only for cost but also for quality of care, so it is important to have a basic understanding of the issues involved. A brief review is then given of the performance of managed care plans relative to traditional fee-for-service. The next section addresses two key policy issues from the perspective of the Medicare program. A final section offers a summary and recommendations for future work.

DEFINITIONS OF MANAGED CARE

The term *health maintenance organization* (HMO) has a generally accepted definition in the research literature and in legislation with respect to the various federal and state programs that regulate HMOs. Usually, it involves a health plan that accepts responsibility for the delivery of a predetermined range of necessary medical services to an enrolled population. HMOs rely minimally on financial incentives such as deductibles to constrain the use of services, although copayments (e.g., $10 per visit), are common. HMOs generally have a set of providers to deliver these services and often do not cover care received from outside providers, unless the plan refers the enrollees there. Many sponsors for enrollees, such as the employer or public agency, require that enrollees be able to choose among various HMOs and possibly a fee-for-service option. The HMO may use a variety of financial and other mechanisms to encourage or compel its providers to keep medical care costs within budget.

Managed care is a much broader and less well-defined concept. Its use often includes and sometimes primarily means HMOs, although it usually also includes systems that may not meet the specific regulatory requirements of certain public agencies. Thus, Medicare can contract with both HMOs and competitive medical plans (CMPs), which may meet different requirements but function similarly to HMOs. From the perspective of the public and many health care providers (a term I use to include hospitals, physicians, and other health professionals), managed care often covers almost any financial arrangement that influences the traditional patient-provider relationship. The idealized view of the traditional relationship assumes care can be obtained from any licensed provider and that a third-party insurer will reimburse the costs with little oversight other than sanctions for outright fraud or refusal to pay the full amount of excessively high fees. This broader view includes situations in which a payer might require prior approval for a proposed procedure or hospital admission or is willing to pay fees that are markedly below "usual" rates.

In this context, one might consider the current fee-for-service Medicare plan to be a type of managed care. Under the prospective payment system

(PPS) implemented in 1983 using diagnosis related groups (DRGs), Medicare pays hospitals a fixed amount for each inpatient stay based on the patient's diagnoses, rather than the costs incurred. Medicare sets the payment levels externally, without negotiation, and thus the hospital has strong incentives to limit the use of extra tests or procedures and to encourage the patient's discharge at the earliest possible time. Since 1992, physician fees under Medicare have been based on the resource based relative value system (RBRVS), which is designed to reflect the costs of various activities and adjusted malpractice and local rent costs. In some instances, these fees are markedly lower than what certain physicians may have been charging. Furthermore, physicians have strong incentives to accept these fees as payment in full and not "balance bill." Currently, most physicians who serve Medicare beneficiaries are participating providers under Medicare and have thus agreed to the fee schedule (Physician Payment Review Commission, 1997). Medicare also contracts with peer review organizations (PROs) to review the patterns of care offered by health professionals and hospitals to ensure that they are maintaining quality standards and rendering appropriate services (see chapter 15). From the provider's perspective, this amounts to a substantial degree of management in contrast to the "good old days." While fee-for-service (FFS) Medicare maintains the patient's individual freedom to choose a provider, the pressures to discharge patients early from the hospitals are pervasive nonetheless.

While the data presented below focus on HMOs or similar entities with whom Medicare may have contracts, patients' and providers' perceptions may well be colored by experiences with other types of arrangements, including some that are now considered FFS Medicare. These issues may be especially important for the more subjective aspects of managed care. We tend to assess current experiences through the comparative lens of "what used to be" and not necessarily "what currently is."

ENROLLMENTS AND PATTERNS OF COVERAGE

Nationally, roughly 53.5 million people are enrolled in HMOs (about 44 million in "pure" HMOs and approximately 9.5 million in point-of-service plans). Among the Medicare population, only 14% were enrolled in HMOs in 1997, and the growth rate has been extraordinary—a 41% increase in Medicare risk contract enrollment from December 1994 to January 1996 (U.S. Department of Health and Human Services, Health Care Financing Administration, 1996). We should, however, place these enrollment figures in context, especially in terms of the overall structure of the Medicare program.

Many people view Medicare as *the* health insurance program for the elderly, but it is both more and less than that. On the one hand, Medicare provides coverage for many nonelderly disabled persons and those eligible under the End Stage Renal Disease Program (ESRD). Disabled and ESRD beneficiaries accounted for 12.6% of the Medicare population in 1996 and, because of the greater medical needs of these groups, a substantially larger fraction of total expenditures (U.S. Department of Health and Human Services, Health Care Financing Administration, 1996). On the other hand, Medicare has important limitations in benefits for the elderly, including substantial deductibles and copayments and no coverage for outpatient pharmaceuticals—an important issue for older persons. Medicare also requires a monthly premium for Part B services (largely outpatient physician services), which, while heavily subsidized, is unaffordable for the poor. Thus, low-income people may be "dually eligible" for Medicare and Medicaid coverage, which combine to cover the premiums, copayments, and deductibles. Furthermore, the Medicaid part often covers services, such as outpatient drugs, more extensively. Those not eligible for Medicaid often obtain supplemental insurance either individually or through their current or past employer. In 1993 only 9% of the aged beneficiaries had FFS Medicare coverage only. Thirty-one percent were covered by employer-sponsored supplemental insurance, 32% by individually purchased supplemental insurance, 8% by employer and individually purchased supplemental insurance, and 13% by Medicaid; 7% were in HMOs (U.S. Department of Health and Human Services, Health Care Financing Administration, 1996).

We should also understand the context in which enrollment in Medicare HMOs occurs. The Medicare program has two arrangements for contracting with HMOs: cost- and risk-based contracts. The cost-based contracts, which cover 10% of Medicare HMO enrollees, allow the HMO to bill Medicare as if it were a fee-for-service plan. Risk-based contracts, which cover the remaining 90%, require the HMO to offer the full set of Medicare-covered services without additional payments from Medicare for individual services. Medicare pays the plan a fixed premium, currently set at 95% of the adjusted average per capita cost (AAPCC), which is supposed to approximate what FFS beneficiaries in the local area would cost the Medicare program. Whether this rate is correct is a very controversial policy question, as discussed below. At this point, it is important to know that the premium level is set by a formula determined by the Health Care Financing Administration (HCFA) that was developed to cover the basic Medicare benefit package. An HMO may choose to forgive all or part of the normally required Part B premiums, the deductibles, and copayments, and may even add other noncovered benefits, such as outpatient pharmaceuticals. In fact, if the HMO's costs are lower than the HCFA payment,

HCFA requires the HMO to add extra benefits or lower beneficiary payments so that the HMO's profit margin for Medicare beneficiaries does not exceed that for other enrollees.

In 1996 95% of risk contract plans offered coverage for an annual physical (not a covered benefit under FFS Medicare), 86% offered immunizations, and 60% offered outpatient prescription drug coverage. Ninety-four plans offered prescription drug benefits as part of their zero premium plan, sometimes with coverage up to $1,500 (Zarabozo, Taylor, & Hicks, 1996). Overall, 63% of enrollees paid no additional monthly premium, and only 18% paid $40 per month or more for their HMO coverage (Lamphere, Neuman, Langwell, & Sherman, 1997). Thus, the vast majority of older HMO enrollees receive a broader benefit package at substantially lower cost than they would with a Medicare supplemental plan.

Even though enrollment of the Medicare population in HMOs is increasing, its spread across the nation is uneven. Forty percent of all risk contract enrollees are in California and Florida. The bottom 23 states account for a total of only 5% of all enrollees. This concentration is not merely a reflection of the relative location of Medicare eligibles. In 1996 about a quarter of beneficiaries had no managed care plan available, and of those living in areas where plans were available, the average enrollment rate was 11% (Henry J. Kaiser Family Foundation, 1997a). In 6 states, over 25% of the Medicare population is in risk contract plans, while in 18 states 1% or less of the population is in such plans. In some counties, the proportion of Medicare beneficiaries in HMOs exceeds 35%.

Much less is known about the nature of the HMOs that enroll the Medicare population, but again we see a picture of high concentration, as 20 plans account for 55% of all enrollment, and five plans account for 30% (Zarabozo et al., 1996). Furthermore, while the classic group and staff model plans, such as Kaiser and Group Health, have substantial enrollments, most of the new growth (except for conversion from cost to risk contracts) has occurred in plans with broader networks of physicians and hospitals. This means that, in many instances, a physician will have a mix of patients with fee-for-service and HMO coverage, often from multiple HMO plans.

This enrollment pattern has several important implications. First, because the standard FFS Medicare package, although universal, has important gaps and financial burdens, those who do not have Medicaid eligibility have a strong incentive to obtain supplemental insurance. For some, this is made available at no cost by their current or former employer. (Recall that Medicare eligibility is age-related, except for the disabled and ESRD beneficiaries. For those who are actively employed, private coverage bears the first responsibility for payment, and Medicare is a secondary payer; most employers design a retirement health package that merely supplements Medicare.) A substantial fraction of the Medicare population pays out-of-pocket premiums to purchase supplemental plans. The broader coverage offered by many HMOs, often with no extra premium cost, is thus an attractive inducement to enroll. For this reason, many Medicare HMO enrollees may have joined not because they like HMOs and their style of care, but because they offer a much less expensive way to fill the gaps in FFS Medicare coverage.

Second, the high concentration of Medicare beneficiaries in certain areas means that average performance assessments of HMOs may be reflecting just a few plans and localities. If there is reason to suspect that these plans and areas are unusual, then it may be incorrect to generalize their performance to what might occur in other parts of the nation. Put another way, in southern California and southern Florida, Medicare HMO enrollments are very high and cannot increase by a factor of more than 2 or 3 (everyone would be enrolled at that point). In the long run, Medicare HMOs will grow in other geographic areas, even without changes in policy, so past performance may not be a reliable guide to the future.

THE ROLE OF RISK SELECTION

The distribution of medical care expenditures is highly skewed, with a small fraction of the population having very high costs and the vast majority using few or no services in a year. This is true for both Medicare and other populations. Typically, about 10% of the eligible group accounts for 75% of expenditures (Henry J. Kaiser Family Foundation, 1997b). The skewness of medical care costs is one of the principal reasons why health insurance is desirable—it allows risk to be spread over large numbers of persons (Arrow, 1963). However, risk spreading occurs only when the pool of covered persons is not selected on the basis of health risk. The classic problem with individual insurance is that potential enrollees may know they will need medical care, so the insurer is legitimately skeptical of why they want to enroll. Large, employer-based groups do not have this problem, because most people join the company for a job, not because they have a particular medical care need.

The Medicare program offers essentially universal coverage for all eligible people; hence it has ample opportunity to spread risk over large numbers of individuals. However, the individual (and his or her spouse) makes the decision to purchase Medicare supplemental insurance. Because of the potential for adverse selection, that is, the attraction of high-risk enrollees to these plans, it is often made difficult for people with preexisting conditions to purchase Medicare supplemental coverage.

The potential for selection also occurs with people joining Medicare HMOs, but in this case the tools available to the plan to deal with selection are different. Rather than just modifying the copayments and deductibles and thus relying on medical underwriting, an HMO is also able to make the plan less desirable to the very ill by restricting its set of referral physicians and hospitals. It may be able to differentially attract low-risk people by marketing benefits, such as dental coverage or eyeglasses that, while valuable to all, may be of relatively greater importance for healthy enrollees than for the very ill. Plan characteristics such as these may evolve for entirely innocent reasons, such as to offer additional benefits to an enrolled population that was less costly than the AAPCC offered by Medicare. Other features, such as special programs for frail older people, might have the opposite impact of attracting high-risk enrollees. It is more likely, however, that the adverse cost implications of such features would lead to the modification or even to the demise of the plan due to noncompetitive costs.

Certain features of Medicare enhance the importance of potential risk selection. First, the population covered—the elderly and disabled—tend to have greater medical care needs in general, so the choice of plan and provider is more salient than is likely to be the case for the rest of the population. Second, substantial gaps in FFS Medicare coverage make it medically important for beneficiaries to consider a Medicare supplemental policy or HMO coverage. Most importantly, Medicare's rules, while designed to protect the beneficiary, encourage risk selection nonetheless. Medicare beneficiaries are allowed to disenroll from an HMO with 30 days' notice, whereas most employer-sponsored plans allow plan switching only once a year. Also, HMOs do not enroll groups of seniors, as they do for employers. Rather, they recruit individuals, so it is not surprising that they may choose to do so at shopping malls, where patrons tend to be healthy.

The presence of risk selection is not a problem if payments to the plans take into account differences in risk. However, Medicare capitation payments are based only on age, sex, disability, Medicaid disability, the institutionalization status of the beneficiaries, and the AAPCC. Numerous studies demonstrate that these variables account for a very small fraction of the variation in the actual cost of medical care (Ash, Porell, Gruenberg, Sawitz, & Beiser, 1989). More important than the low explanatory power is the evidence that many HMOs enroll people at below-average risk of health care utilization (Eggers, 1980; Pear, 1997).

The capitation rate's inadequate accounting for risk differences has several important implications. One is that instead of saving 5% relative to FFS payments for people enrolled in HMOs, Medicare may actually be paying HMOs more than it would pay providers if the HMOs' enrollees had remained in FFS (Physician Payment Review Commission, 1997). We examine the desirability of this differential in the section below on policy issues. The more serious implication is much more subtle. Remember that one possible method for avoiding high-risk people is to have a more limited set of subspecialists and referral centers, or to make access to available resources more difficult in the hope that high users of care will switch back to FFS. Such strategies may result in lower quality of care for enrollees, particularly those with expensive chronic conditions. Poor quality of care for people with occasional acute problems is likely to result in more obvious quality problems and higher costs because poor quality care for acute conditions is often more expensive in the long run.

PERFORMANCE OF HMOS FOR MEDICARE BENEFICIARIES

A recent review summarizes the published literature on HMO performance from 1986 through 1996 (Miller & Luft, 1994a, 1994b, 1997). This section will highlight the findings that are most relevant to understanding Medicare and HMOs. We should note that, due to data collection and publication lags, the most recent data included in any of the papers reviewed is from 1994, and the vast majority of the evidence predates that by several years. Furthermore, the medical care system plausibly has become more competitive and cost-conscious since 1993, so some of these results may have limited bearing on current, let alone future, performance of plans.

On various measures of resource use, such as hospital admission, days, length of stay, and overall expenditures, the evidence is somewhat mixed, but the strongest evidence supports the view that HMOs use fewer resources than FFS plans use.

Measures of enrollee satisfaction generally indicate much higher ratings for HMOs than for FFS with respect to the financial aspects of the plans and generally lower satisfaction with the nonfinancial aspects, such as the technical and interpersonal quality of care. Interestingly, lower-income enrollees, including those with Medicare-Medicaid coverage, seemed to prefer HMOs even with respect to the nonfinancial aspects of coverage (Lurie, Christianson, Finch, & Moscovice, 1994). In part, this may reflect the fact that many physicians are unwilling to accept FFS Medicaid payments, so the broader access offered by HMOs is seen as a positive aspect.

The single most common dimension of HMO performance addressed in the recent literature has been the quality of care, which reflects increasing concern about this issue. In some instances, quality of care was significantly better for Medicare beneficiaries enrolled in HMOs than for those in FFS—for example, for patients admitted to intensive care units (Angus et al., 1996) and for early detection of various cancers (Riley, Potosky, Lubitz, & Brown, 1994). Many studies reflected quality of care that was better on some measures and worse on others. Other studies showed a preponderance of findings indicating worse quality of care in HMOs. Some of these focused only on older persons (Manton, Newcomer, Lowrimore, Vertrees, & Harrington, 1993; Shaughnessy, Schlenker, & Hittle, 1994), while others covered a broader population (Ware, Bayliss, Rogers, Kosinski, & Tarlov, 1996).

Two preliminary patterns are emerging in these findings. The first is that, overall, the results with respect to quality of care are surprisingly balanced, with equal numbers of findings favorable and unfavorable to HMOs. If one expected that the pressures for cost containment would jeopardize quality, then the examples of better quality in HMOs provide strong contrary evidence. On the other hand, if one hoped that HMOs would be able to coordinate care to improve outcomes, the evidence suggests that this is a goal not yet achieved.

Second, some suggest that HMOs are better at handling acute problems and the detection of disease through periodic screening than they are at dealing with complicated chronic conditions. There may be many reasons for this tentative observation; however, this is what one might predict given what we know about HMOs, especially in the context of the Medicare program. As discussed in the preceding section, the structure of the Medicare program enhances risk selection. Even if a plan did not try to get rid of high-risk enrollees, it would face financial disaster by developing visible high-quality programs to take care of the chronically ill. Once the superior performance of such programs were known, Medicare beneficiaries would flock to them, but payments would still be based on the average costs of people in their AAPCC cell, not on the AAPCC plus the extra costs associated with chronic conditions. Thus, superior quality of care is "punished" by the current payment system. Likewise, the absence of good, routinely available measures of quality makes it impossible to sanction any but the most egregious examples of poor quality of care, in either FFS or HMO settings.

POLICY ISSUES

A wide range of policy issues concern the role of managed care plans in the Medicare program. However, we will focus on two major ones: ensuring quality of care and setting appropriate payment levels for health plans. In addressing these, it is important to distinguish two different perspectives that might be relevant to the decision-maker. The first recognizes

Medicare as a program that has high political visibility and needs to be managed in a responsible way. This perspective seeks to protect the integrity of the overall program but does not view managed care as a major tool to either reshape the health care system or markedly change the cost or structure of Medicare. In a sense, this more passive perspective holds to the principle of noninterference in the original Medicare legislation but also recognizes that managed care is making rapid inroads in the employed population and in Medicaid programs, and Medicare will have to adapt to that reality.

The second perspective sees managed care as a valuable tool for achieving other objectives. These might include lowering the federal cost of Medicare below what would be achieved under a more passive policy; they might even extend to using Medicare's clout to reshape the larger health care system. The first of the two goals under this activist perspective would be to stand by the general mandate to prudently manage Medicare expenditures. The second would be more far-reaching.

From either perspective, Medicare should be concerned about the quality of care provided to Medicare beneficiaries in managed care plans, just as it should be concerned about quality in fee-for-service. Medicare should also attempt to pay managed care plans "fair premiums" for the benefits they provide. What exactly a "fair premium" should be and how it should be determined is a complex issue that transcends the scope of this chapter, but we will briefly touch upon it. The different perspectives (passive vs. active) will influence how one chooses to measure the benefits of managed care.

Quality of Care

It is a political reality that the Medicare program will be held responsible for the quality of care that it purchases. In 1990 the Institute of Medicine completed an extensive study, *A Strategy for Quality Assurance in Medicare*, that offered the following definition of quality of care:

> Quality of care is the degree to which health services for individuals and populations increase the likelihood of desired health outcomes and are consistent with current professional knowledge. (Institute of Medicine, 1990, p. 21)

A key aspect of this definition is that it focuses not just on the technical quality of the services rendered but also on their appropriateness, from both a medical and a patient perspective. It also recognizes the need for a population-based focus, so a system that offers the very best to only a few may be less desirable than a system that offers somewhat less, but ensures coverage of a broader population and reaches out to those who otherwise would not get services. Finally, the definition recognizes that not all interventions work as well as one would hope, and thus high-quality care will increase the likelihood of desired health outcomes, although this may not happen in each individual case.

Two important issues arise in assessing the quality of care in managed care settings and in FFS. The first stems from the different incentives in the two systems. The fixed budget held by managed care plans creates an incentive to provide fewer services, while FFS offers incentives for providers to order and deliver more. Thus, one would be tempted to focus primarily on underuse in managed care and overuse in FFS. However, the situation may be more complex than it seems. Most managed care plans offer more comprehensive coverage and a broader range of benefits than standard FFS Medicare. Ample evidence suggests that the deductibles and copayments in FFS Medicare help to constrain medical care use. The absence of certain types of coverage, such as for outpatient prescriptions, is also a factor. This means that if one were to compare managed care enrollees with those in FFS Medicare, there would be incentives within the plan to constrain use, but incentives for the beneficiary to increase use.

Two implications emerge from these countervailing pressures. The first is that the comparison group is unclear. Remember that a mere 9% of Medicare-aged beneficiaries have FFS Medicare–only coverage; the vast majority have purchased supplemental coverage, either by themselves, through an employer, or through a government agency. Yet half of all Medicare HMO enrollees pay nothing extra for their enhanced benefits. Should the quality of their care be compared with that of the FFS Medicare–only people, or should it be compared with that of those who have purchased supplemental coverage, often at substantially higher cost? Thus, if one is concerned that managed care plans limit medical care use, should this be in comparison with a Medicare plan that costs the same and has high copayments, which also reduce use? The notion of context is important; when *Consumer Reports* evaluates automobiles, for instance, they compare cars within the same general price range, rather than Chevrolets vs. Mercedes.

The second point is more subtle, but it relates to the previous observation. People (other than economists) generally do not perceive price as a "rationing" device; they reserve the notion of rationing to situations in which goods or services are allocated in other ways. The mere fact that managed care plans largely eliminate the financial barriers to care may make people *feel* that they are denied more things. For example, an HMO enrollee is likely to be quite angry about a plan's denial of a referral for a simple consultation, even though the enrollee could go to the specialist and pay out of pocket. With FFS coverage and a $200 deductible, the same visit might also be entirely out of pocket, but the person is less likely to be angry. Were the lack of the consultation to cause a delay in diagnosis, this would be seen as a quality failure if the patient were in managed care, but not if the patient were in FFS. An evenhanded assessment of quality will have to address these conceptual issues in a creative way.

The second important complication in assessing quality arises from the different types of data collected in the two settings. FFS Medicare is claims-based and therefore generates detailed bills for all the services rendered, but this information is much less complete with respect to diagnoses and the status of the patient. Some HMOs have detailed encounter and electronic medical record data, which is typically better in terms of lab test results and diagnoses but less detailed in terms of the minor procedures performed. Some HMOs capitate their medical groups and receive very little information, and even when they do, the information is less than optimally consistent across groups.

Managed care plans now routinely report to employers measures of their quality as defined in the Health Plan Employer Data Information Set (HEDIS). While this is an important step forward, these data have received criticism for focusing on a narrow range of quality measures (Epstein, 1995) that are weighted heavily toward preventive activities, such as screening for breast cancer. A new version of HEDIS has been developed that, for the first time, focuses on the Medicare population (in addition to populations covered by commercial plans and Medicaid); plans were required to report 1996 data by mid-1997. In general, these approaches help maintain a public health/prevention focus for plans.

Measuring other aspects of quality is likely to be more difficult, both because the science of quality assessment is less developed and, perhaps more importantly, because the lack of risk adjustment is a financial disincentive for plans to really excel in the care of very sick, chronically ill enrollees. Thus, while the risk adjustment question is clearly on the policy agenda for the near future (see below), the policy focus is on the cost to the program. In fact, a more compelling case for risk adjustment might lie in its impact on the incentives for quality of care.

If Medicare can implement quality monitoring systems that focus on the care of the chronically and seriously ill, which implies the use of data systems that work not only for those in HMOs but also for those in FFS, then beneficial effects will likely extend to the *overall* quality of care. Recalling that 10% of the enrolled population accounts for 75% of expenditures, such a targeted approach may have a major impact on both the quality and cost of care for all and thus meet some of the goals of those with an activist perspective who see Medicare policy as an effector on overall system change, rather than on a narrower set of goals.

Setting Payment Levels for Health Plans

Most observers agree that the current methodology for setting premiums to be paid managed care plans is less than optimal. In some parts of the nation, the payments are so low that few plans are willing to take on risk contracts. In other areas, the AAPCC is so high that plans can offer extensive benefit packages with no extra premium. Payments also may vary markedly from one county to the next, in ways that appear to be arbitrary. The most important policy issues relate to risk adjustment and who should benefit from enrolling in a managed care plan.

The risk adjustment issues are conceptually straightforward but technically complex. Ideally, one should pay plans an amount that reflects the risk mix of their enrollees. The AAPCC was designed to do this but is inadequate to the task, because an AAPCC cell may contain a wide range of risk. Also, the structure and operation of HMOs allow, and sometimes foster, risk selection. Various proposals would apply new risk assessment measures to capture the mix of illness among enrollees (Ash et al., 1989).

A mixed approach would blend fixed capitation payments with FFS reimbursement of plans (Newhouse, 1994; Newhouse, Manning, Keeler, & Sloss, 1989). Another approach would allow plans to exclude from their risk-based payment, yet still take care of, a small fraction of their enrollees who are most likely to be high cost (van Barneveld, van Vliet, & van de Ven, 1996; van de Ven, & van Vliet, 1992). Still another approach would implement supplemental payments for very high-cost conditions, along with detailed clinical information systems to monitor quality of care (Luft & Dudley, 1997).

Regardless of the particular approach taken, the intent would be to pay more to plans that have a high proportion of potentially high-cost people and pay less to plans with relatively healthy people. Unlike the current situation in which plans have strong incentives to not attract the very ill, with appropriate risk-adjusted payments, plans might actually find it beneficial to attract the very ill. Developing a method to save 10% of the cost associated with people having medical costs of $40,000 a year yields much more than saving 10% on the relatively healthy, who cost very little and whose minimal needs are often unavoidable.

Other issues that will have to be addressed in setting the level of risk-adjusted payments are more obscure, such as the geographic variability in payments, and how to account for the costs of graduate medical education that are currently built into the FFS Medicare payments. A larger, more philosophic issue arises from the complex relationship between Medicare and the need for supplemental benefits. Currently, if managed care plans can care for their enrollees at less than the AAPCC level, they must return those savings to the beneficiary in extra benefits or lower premiums or copayments. In essence, the enrollees are able to convert a fixed amount of money into broader benefits and lower out-of-pocket costs relative to Medicare alone. Put another way, they are able to get the financial coverage akin to Medicare supplemental insurance without paying the going rate for such coverage. This additional benefit, however, comes at the price of a more restricted choice of providers and perhaps other limitations.

This leads one to ask, should the risk-adjusted payment, regardless of its method of determination, be at the level that would cover only the cost of Medicare without supplemental coverage, or should it cover this broader set of benefits, recognizing that the patient may be giving up something of value in joining the HMO? If the lower level were chosen, few people would join HMOs, since they would pay separately for supplemental benefits yet have restricted choice. On the other hand, some may argue that allowing beneficiaries to reap those extra benefits at no extra cost adds to the federal expense. Geographic equity issues also arise if not everyone has a managed care plan available in their locality; income equity issues arise if not everyone can equally afford supplemental premiums.

Another perspective views managed care plans as competitive market forces. A recent review (Miller & Luft, 1997) identified several studies of the effects of managed care on local medical care use and costs. Many of these studies observed that resource use declined or costs grew less rapidly in areas with heavy managed care presence. Thus, the competitive pressure of managed care may change the behavior of all providers, helping to contain costs. This may occur even when the performances of managed care and FFS providers differ very little. If other studies bear out these findings, then one may wish to encourage the growth of managed care not just because it lowers costs for those enrollees, but because it changes the performance of the overall system. (Current evidence on this "spillover" effect concentrates on cost issues, but quality may also be affected. The challenge will be to structure the incentives and quality monitoring to ensure that the competitive effect is to lower cost and raise quality, rather than vice versa.) From this perspective, offering inducements to Medicare beneficiaries to join managed care plans may be worthwhile, as this may help transform the overall system in a desired way. While "bribes" clearly would be inappropriate, allowing plans to offer additional benefits within the basic Medicare premium level, as is done now, may be quite reasonable and would not involve a change in underlying policy. The beneficial spillover effects, however, may help counter the arguments of those who feel that even an appropriately risk-adjusted payment to managed care plans might be too high.

SUMMARY

This chapter intends to set the stage for further thinking about the role of managed care in the Medicare program, recognizing that this is a rapidly changing area. It does not address some policy questions that may be included in a more comprehensive discussion of managed care for Medicare beneficiaries. Such questions include whether Medicare benefits for home care, pharmaceuticals, and other services might be expanded or modified; the impact of block grants to states for Medicaid costs, and how that will affect dually eligibles; and societal perspectives on the right to die and end-of-life care. We omitted these issues largely because so little is known, either about their current impact or about how the Medicare program will change.

Instead, we have chosen to focus on some underlying issues, in particular, the importance of considering Medicare in the context of other programs for older or disabled persons and in the context of the larger medical care environment. It is misleading to focus only on FFS Medicare without recognizing that less than 10% of the Medicare beneficiaries rely solely on this program; their utilization, cost, and quality of care are shaped by their coverage. Likewise, the heavy concentration of managed care enrollment in a few geographic areas means that the lessons we draw from existing plan performance may have little bearing on a much broader future enrollment pattern.

The published evidence on the performance of managed care plans is surprisingly balanced in terms of satisfaction and quality. This contrasts with the media coverage, which typically focuses on problems of managed care. The conflicting perspectives may be due to the older data on which the published studies are based or may simply reflect that the media do not find interesting stories of "no problems." (How often does one read an article about the jet plane that took off fully loaded, had a smooth flight, and landed on schedule?) Not all the research finds HMOs better or less costly.

Perhaps a more important message is that the current system is not well designed to encourage good performance by managed care plans. The payment to plans set by HCFA does not take into account differential risk, resulting in overpayments to plans with lower than average risk. The desire for enrollee protections led to beneficiaries' right to change plans on 30-day notice, but this exacerbates the selection problem. More important than the overpayment of plans is the disincentive for plans to develop high-quality programs to care for people with expensive chronic conditions. Even without systems to encourage plans to want the sickest enrollees, the absence of sensitive measures of quality and incentives for good care means that managed care will, if only by default, focus on cost, rather than quality. Moreover, the easy ability to switch coverage and the rapidly changing policy environment favor plans with short- rather than long-term perspectives on performance.

In the debates surrounding Medicare and managed care, there is too much attention on a search for villains, among both policymakers and health plans. A different perspective emerges from a more complete understanding of how Medicare fits in the larger environment and of how relatively obscure issues, such as risk adjustment, influence plans and enrollees. Increased attention to some of these policy details may allow the creation of a more effective and efficient Medicare program in the future.

REFERENCES

Angus, D. C., Linde-Zwirble, W. T., Sirio, C. A., Rotondi, A. J., Chelluri, L., Newbold, R. C., III, Lave, J. R., & Pinsky, M. R. (1996). The effect of managed care on ICU length of stay: Implications for Medicare. *Journal of the American Medical Association, 276,* 1075–1082.

Arrow, K. J. (1963). Uncertainty and the welfare economics of medical care. *American Economic Review, 53,* 941–973.

Ash, A., Porell, F., Gruenberg, L., Sawitz, E., & Beiser, A. (1989). Adjusting Medicare capitation payments using prior hospitalization data. *Health Care Financing Review, 10,* 17–29.

Eggers, P. (1980). Risk differentials between Medicare beneficiaries enrolled and not enrolled in an HMO. *Health Care Financing Review, 2,* 91–99.

Epstein, A. E. (1995). Performance reports on quality—prototypes, problems, and prospects. *New England Journal of Medicine, 333,* 57–61.

Henry J. Kaiser Family Foundation. (1995). *Medicare chart book* (fig. 17). Washington, DC: Author.

Henry J. Kaiser Family Foundation. (1997a). *Medicare chart book* (fig. 27). Washington, DC: Author.

Henry J. Kaiser Family Foundation. (1997b). *Medicare chart book* (fig. 18). Washington, DC: Author.

Institute of Medicine. (1990). *Medicare: A strategy for quality assurance* (Vol. 1). Washington, DC: National Academy Press.

Lamphere, J. A., Neuman, P., Langwell, K., & Sherman, D. (1997). The surge in Medicare managed care: An update. *Health Affairs, 16,* 127–133.

Luft, H. S., & Dudley, R. A. (1997). (Revised and resubmitted).

Luft, H. S., & Dudley, R. A. (1997). Encouraging health plans to provide excellent care for very sick people. (Revised and resubmitted).

Lurie, N., Christianson, J., Finch, M., & Moscovice, I. (1994). The effects of capitation on health and functional status of the Medicaid elderly. *Annals of Internal Medicine, 120,* 506–511.

Manton, K. G., Newcomer, R., Lowrimore, G. R., Vertrees, J. C., & Harrington, C. (1993). Social/health maintenance organization and fee-for-service health outcomes over time. *Health Care Financing Review, 15,* 173–202.

Miller, R. H., & Luft, H. S. (1994a). Managed care plan performance since 1980: A literature analysis. *Journal of the American Medical Association, 271,* 1512–1519.

Miller, R. H., & Luft, H. S. (1994b). Managed care plans: Characteristics, growth, and premium performance. *Annual Review of Public Health, 15,* 437–459.

Miller, R. H., & Luft, H. S. (1997). Does managed care lend to better or worse quality of care? *Health Affairs, 16,* 7–25.

Newhouse, J. P. (1994). Patients at risk: Health reform and risk adjustment. *Health Affairs, 13,* 132–146.

Newhouse, J. P., Manning, W. G., Keeler, E. B., & Sloss, E. M. (1989). Adjusting capitation rates using objective health measures and prior utilization. *Health Care Financing Review, 10,* 41–54.

Pear, R. (1997, March 29). Cut urged in Medicare money to H.M.O.'s. *New York Times,* p. 10.

Physician Payment Review Commission. (1997). *Annual report to Congress.* Washington, DC.

Riley, G. F., Potosky, A. L., Lubitz, J. D., & Brown, M. L. (1994). Stage of cancer at diagnosis for Medicare HMO and fee-for-service enrollees. *American Journal of Public Health, 84,* 1598–1604.

Shaughnessy, P. W., Schlenker, R. E., & Hittle, D. F. (1994.) Home health care outcomes under capitated and fee-for-service payment. *Health Care Financing Review, 16,* 187–221.

Social Security Act of 1965, Title XVIII, Section 1801.

U.S. Department of Health and Human Services, Health Care Financing Administration. (1996). Profiles of Medicare. Washington, DC.

van Barneveld, E. M., van Vliet, R. C. J. A., & van de Ven, W. P. M. M. (1996). Mandatory high-risk pooling: A means for reducing the incentives for cream skimming. *Inquiry, 33,* 133–143.

van de Ven, W. P. M. M., & van Vliet, R. C. J. A. (1992). How can we prevent cream skimming in a competitive health insurance market? The great challenge for the 90's. *Developments in Health Economic Public Policy, 1,* 23–46.

Ware, J. E., Bayliss, M. S., Rogers, W. H., Kosinski, M., & Tarlov, A. R. (1996). Differences in 4-year health outcomes for elderly and poor, chronically ill patients treated in HMO and fee-for-service systems: Results from the Medical Outcomes Study. *Journal of the American Medical Association, 276,* 1039–1047.

Zarabozo, C., Taylor, C., & Hicks, J. (1996). Medicare managed care: Numbers and trends. *Health Care Financing Review, 17,* 243–261.

19

Necessary Changes in the Infrastructure of Health Systems

George Halvorson

Organized care. Coordination. Integration. Systems-based approaches. Those themes are prevalent throughout this book. Providers and care-givers generally agree that older people's health needs are best served when all parts of the system work together and align toward dual goals: preventing illness and injury among older people and coordinating care when care is eventually needed. But there is no agreement on how best to reconfigure our current care delivery and financing systems to respond to the unique needs of our aging population. That disagreement stems, in large part, from the fact that our current system is so fragmented in both care delivery and care financing that the challenges of integration seem almost insurmountable (see chapter 16).

All parties agree that our current health care system does not approach care on a systematic basis. We do not have multidisciplinary teams of providers focusing as teams on the health of a population—in this dis-cussion, older people. Instead, our system approaches care as a series of unrelated events; our providers function with minimal teamwork and almost no sense of care continuity between our care sites or even incidents of care or treatment.

Nor do we have payment approaches that reward or even encourage coordination of care. For example, Medicare and Medicaid have different regulations about what is covered and different criteria for payments to providers. Neither program pays providers for preventive care that would encourage better health among older persons. The government, as the major purchaser of health care services for older people, does not track or reward outcomes of care, it merely crudely pays for procedures, with no focus on the effectiveness of the treatment.

Therefore, our current approach contains little or no organized and systematic emphasis on prevention, comparative care outcomes, or value-based market competition between providers on the basis of cost or excellence. Older people are not alone in being treated in the context of a non-system. Our health care system for all patients, not just older Americans, needs to be changed. There are some unique aspects of care for older people, such as the amount of care purchased by the government versus private payers, but in reality, moving to a more systematic and coordinated approach to care would benefit everyone.

The core changes necessary are (1) an emphasis on measurable quality; (2) caregivers who function as teams, not as separate business units; (3) a prepayment, not a per-procedure payment system; (4) a competitive marketplace, with caregivers organized into teams that compete for patients based on service, quality, and cost; (5) informed consumers who have information about caregivers and are able to "shop" for the providers that best meet their needs; (6) appropriate use of technology; (7) use of prepaid care systems; and (8) information systems that support outcomes and care tracking and the use of technology to help physicians and other caregivers improve care.

Older patients would benefit from such systems, just by virtue of more systematic management of their more chronic, ongoing health problems. Unlike younger people, who may have sporadic health care needs, older people are much more likely to need preventive, acute, and chronic care. They would benefit from a system that rewards teams of caregivers, able to offer them coordinated chronic and acute services. They would also benefit from a payment system that rewards providers for improved outcomes and prevention of illness, not just paying them after injuries or illnesses have occurred. They would benefit from competition among providers, who are rewarded for how well they meet the complex challenges of chronic illness. And they would benefit from being able to have a wealth of information about their providers, ranging from which clinics are on bus lines, to which providers have the best outcomes after hip surgery.

Managed care has the potential to offer providers a set of extremely useful tools that could be used to improve both the quality and the outcomes of care for older people. Managed care also, however, has the potential to create a care environment focused excessively on cost control agendas rather than on improved patient care. Which set of outcomes will prevail? Will the older people of the future find themselves in sophisticated, quality-focused, outcomes-based, efficient systems of care? Or will they be in the grips of profit-driven providers and health plans whose motivation is clearly financially based and whose care is built on a platform of rationing and denial rather than on quality, coordination, and improved outcomes?

The system that is developed will be determined in large part by the structure of the senior marketplace that will be created by the federal and state governments over the next few years. For the new market environment to truly benefit older people, it has to be built around quality and value, not simply around efficiency and price. Patients and their families need data about the care system—more sophisticated data than they have ever had—to allow them to become value-based purchasers of care. When consumers have comparative data in hand about the quality, outcomes, satisfaction levels, service levels, accessibility, credentials, and costs of various providers, then they can reward the best providers by choosing to be their patients in an open market environment.

If the market functioned at optimal levels, the sickest patients would be able to select the best providers, and the quality of care would be both known and continuously improved. For that marketplace to exist, it is necessary both to create a data base that facilitates sophisticated consumer choices and to create financing systems that pay more money to the providers who are selected by the sickest patients. Therefore, it makes sense to begin to move our federal programs toward data-based consumer choice models, and it makes equally good sense to create better coordination of the financing of acute and long-term care.

Critics of the value-based market environment contend that data about the quality of care is not yet adequate to serve the purpose of informing consumer choice. There is, in fact, some truth to this assertion. As discussed in chapter 15, the whole area of quality measurement and reporting is in its infancy, and longitudinal, comparative data are not available on many topics. But the process has been started, and a foundation has been laid. Data that are relevant to patients are now being gathered and reported. We now need to build on that foundation to make the data more robust and relevant as quickly as we can.

Ideally, the new marketplace and care environment should reflect the reality that prevention, acute care, chronic care, and long-term care are all part of the same continuum. Although the payment approaches tend to divide these levels of care among Medicare, Medicaid, and personal out-of-pocket expenditures, the best care systems of the future will be organized around the patient, rather than being dictated by segregated payment sources. Data available to consumers need to reflect that entire continuum of care, for example, identifying not only which team of providers has the lowest mortality rate for heart surgery but also which have done the best proactive job of preventing heart attacks in the first place and which have created the greatest patient satisfaction with the care of chronic heart problems. To achieve these goals, care systems need to take a population-based approach to health, thinking like epidemiologists as well as clinicians, to identify the high-impact, high-leverage interventions that are possible in people's lives relative to both preventing disease and minimizing its complications and impact.

To achieve the goal of a coordinated, patient-focused, value-based marketplace, we need to build the new market environment one step at a time, beginning with providing relevant quality data. So, first steps first—we need to create a value-based marketplace for acute care. Then we need to extend that marketplace to the entire continuum of care, using physician-developed, evidence-based clinical guidelines that integrate care rather than separate care. Patients will benefit immensely when we finally make that transition.

To create that type of marketplace, health care organization leaders and CEOs will need to work directly with the purchasers of health care coverage—the employers and public agencies that actually pay for that coverage—to persuade them that a value-based marketplace is both desirable and doable. That marketplace will come about only when it is supported by the payers—and the payers need guidance from health care leaders relative to how that market should be structured and what it can accomplish.

As we prove to patients, providers, and public officials that a competitive provider marketplace is possible—and as we begin to acquaint policymakers with the real quality improvements that come from integrated care teams and an accountable marketplace—those same policymakers who now perpetuate a splintered and uncoordinated set of funding sources will realize the immense positive potential of applying outcomes measurement and value-based consumer choices to the entire spectrum of care. When that happens, the policymakers will begin finally to work with us. Until that level of reporting exists and the value of care coordination is proven, however, the barriers will be defended and maintained.

Index

Page numbers in *italic* indicate figures.
Page numbers followed by "t" indicate tables.